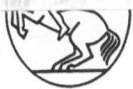

Disorders of Human Communication 8

Edited by G. E. Arnold, F. Winckel, B. D. Wyke
Executive Editor: B. D. Wyke

Wilbur J. Gould
Van L. Lawrence
Surgical Care
of Voice Disorders

With a Contribution
by Nobuhiko Isshiki

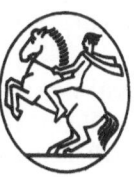

Springer-Verlag Wien New York

Dr. Wilbur J. Gould

Director, Vocal Dynamics Laboratory, Lenox Hill Hospital, New York, N.Y., U.S.A.

Dr. Van L. Lawrence

MacGregor Medical Association, Houston, Tex., U.S.A.

Prof. Dr. Nobuhiko Isshiki

Director, Division of Plastic and Reconstructive Surgery,
School of Medicine, Kyoto University, Kyoto, Japan

With 42 Figures

Library of Congress Cataloging in Publication Data. Gould, Wilbur J. Surgical care of voice disorders. (Disorders of human communication, ISSN 0173-170X; 8.) Bibliography: p. Includes index. 1. Larynx – Surgery. 2. Voice disorders – Surgery. I. Lawrence, Van. II. Isshiki, N. (Nobuhiko) III. Title. IV. Series. [DNLM: 1. Larynx – Surgery. 2. Voice disorders – Surgery. W1 DI762 v. 8 / WV 540 G698s.] RF516.G68. 1984. 617'.533. 83-20058

ISSN 0173 170 X
ISBN-13:978-3-7091-8731-9   e-ISBN-13:978-3-7091-8729-6
DOI: 10.1007/978-3-7091-8729-6

Preface

Contemporary laryngology had its beginnings near the close of the 19th century and is probably best exemplified in the work of Morel McKenzie and of Czermak. Subsequent to their pioneering efforts, another surge of interest could be said to have centered about the efforts of the Chevalier Jacksons in the 1920's. After those bold steps, and for almost 40 years, research in laryngology and interest in laryngology continued, but at considerably and increasingly less intense levels, certainly so far as the otolaryngologist population was concerned. In the 1940's Julius Lempert sparked a renaissance in otologic research, development, and surgery, and exciting new frontiers opened in otology. In our own time, otology remains a large basic and fundamental segment of the otolaryngologic purview, but the flood of new discoveries which followed Lempert, like those which had followed the Jacksons in the 1920's in laryngology, appears to have diminished.

When the authors of this publication made acquaintance in the late 1960's, there were approximately 10 centers in the United States for laryngologic research which could be truly designated as voice research facilities. The senior author was at that time instrumental in formulating the major criteria for laboratories to be so designated.

In the early 1980's interest in laryngology has revived. At a recent meeting it was possible to list over 40 such laboratories which now were known to the authors over a broad geographic sweep, covering the entire United States. That figure did not include the many voice laboratories centered in Japan.

Along with voice research there has been a corresponding growth of interest in laryngeal surgery, as this relates to voice production. Sadly, the authors have shared the unhappy experience of seeing patients in consultation after an injudicious choice of surgical procedures had been made or whose physical management had been less than dexterous.

This publication celebrates the current resurgence of interest in laryngology and details aspects of the authors' experience and philosophy regarding laryngeal surgery and voice production.

May 1984   **The Authors**

Contents

Introduction 1

For most professionals or student professionals who are engaged in caring for individuals who present themselves for help, for diagnosis, or for re-training of the voice as this relates to a particular problem in function of the voice, the need for surgery on a patient's vocal tract should represent failure. There are, of course, a multitude of conditions, situations, circumstances, many of them benign ones as well, over which neither the attendant professional team nor the patient has any etiologic control. People cannot, after all, choose their parentage nor their genetic make-up, and they certainly have no directional say over the vagaries of an embryologic accident occurring previous to their birth. But for many of the problems which beset the vocal tract and which then interfere with its adequate, its appropriate or its ideal functioning, surgery represents the end stage in an ability properly to treat, to diagnose, or even, to cope. In the management of patients with vocal problems there should ideally be a team: a team consisting of a good speech therapist-diagnostician who maintains close rapport with the patient, an involved laryngologist who has his wits about him and his diagnostic acumen sharpened, plus a strongly motivated patient who comprehends his participation in the overall scheme of things as well as his diagnosis and prognosis. This team, then, ought to do fairly well with the satisfactory management, with the satisfactory solution of problems besetting the subject, with most of the more common voice disorders. A requirement for surgery often means that somewhere along the line, one of the team members has faltered, has misdiagnosed, has lost enthusiasm or momentum.

Surgery is still necessary for some voice problems, however, even when the team of patient and therapists possesses all of these attributes, and in full measure. No amount of patient compliance, or speech pathologist-physician-therapist enthusiasm is likely to do much about the ravages of an idiopathic recurrent laryngeal nerve palsy, or the airway obstruction of juvenile laryngeal papillomatosis without the help of vocal tract surgery. But here, too, a purposeful onslaught by a team should bring about the best possible, the best available results.

A word of caution is in order. In many contexts, one of the classical aphorisms is worthy of consideration: the concept of moderation in all things. There are over-enthusiastic patients who take doubled doses of medication hoping to do twice as much good, eagerly committed therapists who are convinced that their own modality of treatment carries with it the quintessential answers to the problem, dextrous, facile surgeons: each of these may view his own area as the definitive one for successful therapy. More often than not, however, successful voice care does indeed represent a combined effort, reached only through the successful inter-relation and inter-reactions of the team members concerned.

This writing addresses itself to some of those vocal tract circumstances which do require surgery as a primary choice for therapy, and will attempt to delineate and outline how the authors think and feel about those different issues which will be mentioned. Some of those issues are both complicated and controversial. An appropriate instrument armamentarium will be mentioned in reasonable detail, as will be the surgical technique in which it is employed, or as we employ it, after those professionals who are concerned have done their very best to be assured of diagnosis, prognosis and the need for surgery. But finally, it should still be stated that for many, many of the more common vocal tract lesions, the authors feel that surgery represents a final court of appeal, and thereby a failure in conventional management either by the patient, or by one of the professionals involved.

This work is not intended only for the neophyte resident in laryngology, to give him an overview of vocal tract surgery. It is not a handbook on vocal tract surgical technique. This work is also intended for the voice practitioner, the therapist/teacher/diagnostician, in the hopes that it will give that person a similar overview of some of the surgical solutions to problems which may trouble or even incapacitate the patient with whom work is undertaken. It is also frankly intended for that person as a vade mecum through some of the tangled thickets of conflicting surgical opinion. Finally, it is hoped that this work, or parts of it, disseminated, and comprehended perhaps with the therapist's assistance, by the intelligent and enthusiastic student/patient, will enable that student/patient to enter into a more informed discussion with his laryngologist about the possible alternatives regarding a choice of surgery or of therapy or both.

Patient Examination: History, Diagnosis, Patient Records 2

A. Patient's Medical History

1. Discussion

It may seem perhaps redundant to say so, but before a surgeon or his assistant does recommend surgery to a patient, there first should be a secure *diagnosis*. Elemental to the procuring of an adequate diagnosis is the taking of a careful history from the patient concerning his illness or his problem. This statement may even seem to resemble those recipes for cooking elephant pie: those which begin with the admonition that first you catch an elephant. A patient's *history* may very well indicate and then even dictate to a great extent, the goals of an approach which will terminate in a surgical procedure. Should the history reflect professional needs of a particular type, in many instances, this may very well result in the choice of a different surgical procedure or in some instances, the abandonment of the recommendation for surgery. More specifically, a person who has chronic hoarseness may well find that the symptom is indeed affecting the proper performance of his job. It may be an indication of an underlying vocal fold pathology such as vocal fold nodules. This same speaker may also have a very high pitched voice which it may be important to correct surgically – a factor of less importance for persons in more isolated occupation such as bookkeeper or as housewife, where quality of voice or tambour of voice may not be of as much relevance as it is in a minister, or a public school teacher.

2. Occupation

Another historical consideration which is of major importance is then that of patient *occupation*. Patient occupation, and the ambient noise levels which will be inherent to that occupation also affect the vocal quality which will be achievable. Since these are factors of major influence, they will probably affect both surgical result and certainly the pre-surgical evaluation. For those persons working in high-background noise environments such as linotypers, boilermakers or public speakers, the surgical requirements are different than are those for persons working in quieter and, therefore, vocally less stressful conditions [48]. Excessive use of voice on the telephone, as in the stock broker, as well as manner of telephone usage (e.g. head position during conversation, use of speaker-phone, intensity of vocal effort required) may have a bearing on the surgical plan.

3. Environmental Factors

Not to be overlooked are the implications of other *environmental factors* on vocal disorders: the climate to which the patient is exposed, whether it be humid, smoggy, dusty or high in altitude. Is the patient a policeman directing traffic in an urban concrete canyon all day long? This will affect voice pathology and selection of therapy. Because of the extreme dryness of a desert place such as Las Vegas, Nevada, requirements for vocal production will be different from those in more humid regions and, accordingly, so must be the therapy and the therapeutic modalities which are chosen for the patient who is placed in such a setting.

4. Considerations of Sex and Age

Historically, the patient's *sex and age* are also major considerations. The maintenance of a female-sounding voice will be a goal in surgery on females just as maintenance of masculine vocal characteristics should be considered when vocal tract surgery is done on a male. The patient's age is important. There are natural variations in tonal quality which are desirable at various ages [49]. The inter-relationship of sex, age, and occupation must also be taken into account. For example, a 24-year old male with an exceedingly high-pitched voice suggesting femininity may be excluded from a desired occupation should it require a deep, masculine, and authoritative voice. A young female receptionist will not benefit from a telephone voice so low in pitch that customers respond to her as "Sir", or "Mister", even though each of those patients functions well from the vocal standpoint without signs of vocal fatigue or of vocal deficit after periods of voice use.

5. Influences of Past History

Another historical factor to be considered here is more general. What has been the patient's recent *symptomatic cause,* and what is the *past general medical history?* Pathology should be considered as to its precise location in time, its duration, and its state of activity, whether static, progressive, or regressive. In static or progressive situations it is more likely that surgical therapy would be considered, while medical therapy would probably be more apt if the condition were regressive. Duration is of great importance, for the presence of the problem for weeks, months, or years will have a direct bearing on considerations of whether to apply medical therapy or directly to initiate surgical procedures. The patient's history of upper respiratory tract surgery (including surgery on sinuses, nasal septum, tonsils and thyroid), as well as a record of localized and chronic infection (including emphysema, bronchitis, asthma, and sinusitis) must also be considered. If the history should show that hoarseness is exaggerated at the time of upper respiratory infection, this may suggest the presence of subglottal polyps – known to be affected by edema resulting from infection and vocal abuse [50]. If this is the case, a direct laryngoscopic examination (discussed in a later section) would be a requisite in order to establish the presence of the possible subglottal pathology. Sinusitis may be a source of vocal problems because so often there is an associated frequent throat clearing which easily may cause chronic laryngitis.

6. Endocrine Influences

Historically, the *endocrine system* must be considered. In the female subject, menstrual history may have a bearing on the problem. This is particularly true for polyps, which can be aggravated by becoming swollen from premenstrual edema. If this is the case, the combination of appropriate speech therapy and appropriate endocrine therapy may correct the menstrual disorder and be a more successful alternative to surgical removal of the polyp. Similarly, thyroid malfunction may be related to a vocal disorder because of the concomitant vocal fold edema associated with that which is often virtually a sub-clinical thyroid hypofunction. Is the patient currently receiving, or has he been receiving androgenic hormone administration for temporary or permanent conditions? In the female subject, a severe dysmenorrhea, an endometriosis, an irregularity of menses, for example, have these been managed by the internist or the gynecologist with androgens? Androgen use in these circumstances is both common and valid in gynecologic practice, and may have far-ranging influences both on the voice, as well as on a proposed surgical plan for a laryngeal problem [51].

7. Birth Control Pill

Elemental in any endocrine consideration are the *influences of the "pill"*. The "pill" currently used for contraceptive purposes or for gynecologic therapy is capable of exerting a powerful influence on the female voice, particularly on the upper range voice. "Pills" usually contain a mixture of the two female hormones: an estrogen, and a progestin [52]. Progestins, owing to their very close biochemical similarity to testosterone (see Fig. 1) can exert a virilizing effect which may be manifested by a loss of the top one or more tones. Should a progestin-dominant medication be necessary for treatment of an underlying gynecologic problem, subsequent laryngeal surgical procedures to affect voice change will certainly be influenced, and may be doomed. At least, historically, the taking for whatever purpose of a "pill" should be noted and its effect on the situation considered.

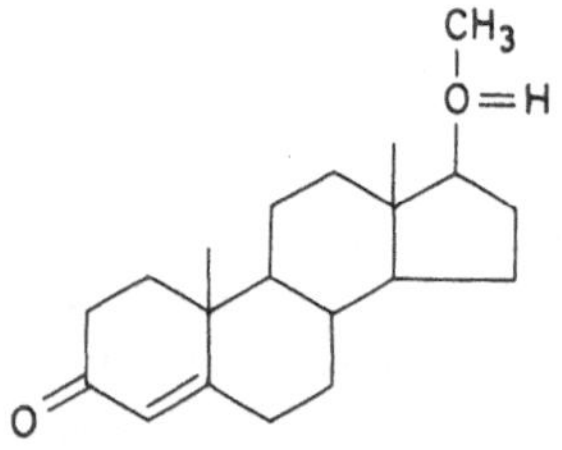

PROGESTERONE

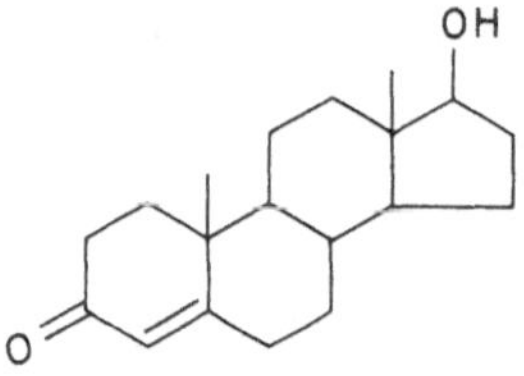

TESTOSTERONE

Fig. 1. Structural formulas for testosterone and progesterone

8. "Recreational" Drugs

Habit patterns may have a great impact on the production of voice pathology as well as on surgical planning. The vast majority of patients with generalized vocal fold polyps demonstrate an edema in Reinke's pouch. Invariably, these patients both smoke and drink liberally, and although the condition may be surgically treated, it promptly will recur if the patient continues these habits. Chronic drug use must also be considered [53]. Does the patient exhibit the vocal fold irritation common among marijuana smokers or does he have the characteristic vocal dryness associated with the use of cocaine? Unusual breath force used with coughing, habitual coughing, or throat-clearing habits can be murderous to a good operative result after vocal polyp removal. Other stressful social habits, such as regular late evening sessions at night clubs, can break down the best surgical results and recreate a vocal fold nodule or tendency to a polypoid condition.

9. Emotions

The general psychological condition, indeed the *emotional factors* manifested by the patient should be evaluated judiciously, cautiously and carefully during the interview. Evidences of excessive tension, or of vocal hesitation in answering certain questions may suggest a psychological disorder, and spontaneous statements by the patient regarding his psychological condition or his view of this condition should be considered. Tense neck muscles and tenderness in the area near the posterior section of the hyoid bone may be other signs indicating muscle tension and possible psychological stress. Psychotherapy sessions, particularly those involving "primal scream" as therapy certainly can cause, and certainly can affect vocal pathology and therapy, and as such should be duly noted. Speech therapists and other voice practitioners are usually neither trained in psychodiagnosis nor in psychotherapy, but when a patient's behaviour appears aberrant enough to make an impression on the historian, that impression is usually worth of serious consideration, and appropriate consultation and/or clarification requested [54].

B. Physical Diagnosis

1. General Diagnostic Evaluations

Again, at the risk of hectoring the reader, it may be said that too few of us really look at our patients. Signs which would suggest pulmonary involvement should be noted: the pale blue gray, the cyanosis in the color of the lips and fingernails for instance, or clubbing of the fingertips. Too seldom do we "lay on hands." We should palpate and feel the neck tissues, examining for neck abnormalities, including cervical nodes and cysts. We may encounter soft masses such as branchial cysts which are congenital and other distortions of the neck such as a thyroglossal cyst or cystic hygroma. Certainly as well, that very laying on of hands has long been known to be of therapeutic value in and of itself. And just as certainly when one is palpating, malposition of the trachea, or any deviation from the midline should be noted.

2. Vocal Dynamics Testing

More complex, and more various diagnostic methodologies may be employed to assess the patient's otolaryngologic condition and need for surgery, and primary among these is vocal dynamics testing [55].

The basic consideration in vocal dynamics functioning relates, of course, to the adequacy of air supply to the sound generator, and this in turn relates to pulmonary function. All of the attributes of pulmonary function need not be studied in this context, but since it is vital that the sound generator itself receive an adequate supply of air with which to create voice, it is essential that some of the parameters of lung air-flow and volume studies be known. There have been many tests for lung and pulmonary air-flow over the past several decades, but perhaps one of the simplest and one of the most effective means of testing this parameter would begin with the use of a spirometer (Fig. 2).

In the use of this test, the subject places the mouthpiece of the breathing tube in his mouth and then on instruction from the technician, the subject breathes in and out. The tube from the mouthpiece is connected with a cylinder suspended from above and placed into a container of water. As the subject exhales, breath passes through the tubing, enters the cylinder which is suspended in water, displaces water and thereby elevates the cylinder. If the cylinder, in turn, be suspended from an overhead point, it is then possible to measure with tracing paper the amount of air which enters and which leaves the cylinder during quiet respiration, forced respiration and so forth. This trace, written and graphed on a sheet of moving paper, is recorded as a

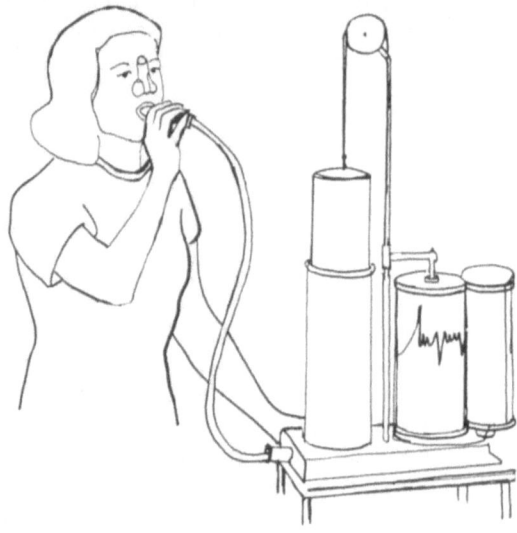

Fig. 2. Spirometer diagram.
(Redrawn from Netter, F.: Spirometry. Ciba Clinical Symposia 27, 11)

spirogram. This directly measures the volume of air inspired or expired during each respiratory cycle, and that volume is referred to as Tidal Volume (TV). Other measures which are of interest in this particular study include the Minute Variation (MV) which is the amount of air inspired and expired in one minute of normal respiration. If the subject is breathing quietly, at the end of expiration, there will be a quantity of air which remains behind in the lung substance and bronchial tree. The amount of air which can be forcefully expressed after the end of quiet expiration is referred to as the Expiratory Reserve Volume (ERV). If the subject takes a maximal inspiration of air and then forcefully expells from the lungs a maximum volume of gas, that amount is referred to as the Vital Capacity (VC). The maximal amount of gas volume which the subject can inspire from the resting quiet physiologic expiratory level is referred to as the Inspiratory Capacity (IC). Vital capacity in the normal adult will vary from about six liters in the tall adult male to approximately three liters in the adult small female. Vital capacity is also a major determinant of the length of phrase which a subject can speak or sing, and the vital capacity, in turn, will be directly affected by variations in posture, thorax compression or expansion, etc. Ultimately, of course, chest capacity will relate to the pressure applied from below and through the diaphragm by the semi-fluid abdominal contents. The weight of the abdominal contents will have a downward moment when the individual is standing and an upward moment (relative to the thoracic cage) when the individual is reclining (see Fig. 3).

Measurement of other parameters of pulmonary function, however, requires other instrumentation. The volume of gas which remains in the lungs at the end of quiet expiration and the airway resistance are both important factors to consider [56]. Measurement of these attributes is currently

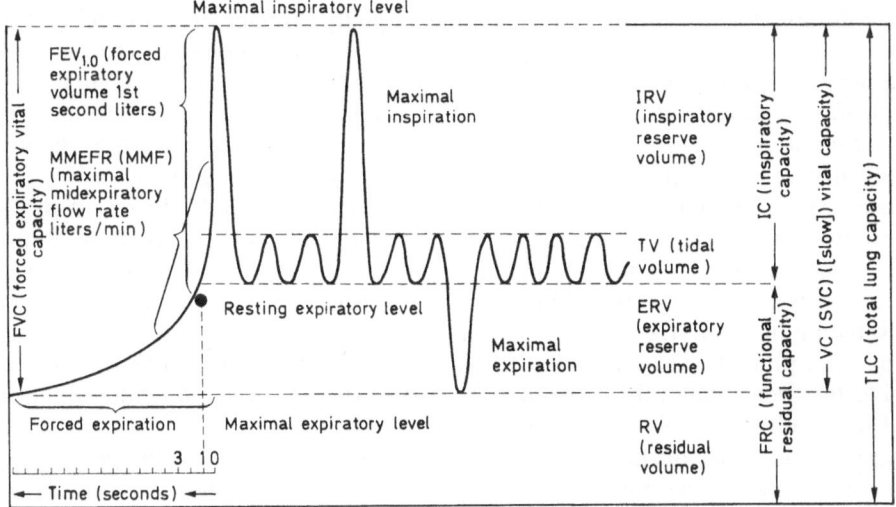

Fig. 3. Pulmonary volumes graph.
(Redrawn from Netter, F.: Spirometry. Ciba Clinical Symposia 27, 11)

accomplished with some form of plethysmograph. While there is a large variety of equipment which is available for plethysmography, the current choice seems to be for some form of fairly firmly fitting tunic which can be worn by the subject and into which are incorporated various sensing devices for pressure changes, volume changes and linear measurement changes in the expired air. The ideal, of course, is that if one is measuring either speech or singing, that one would leave the mouth of the subject unimpaired, and to some extent this is possible with a thoracic tunic plethysmograph. A more accurate (but more troublesome) determination of these same factors can be undertaken if the subject's entire body is placed into a water-filled tank: then there is relatively little encumberance of the thoracic wall movements or of the abdominal wall movements. Probably a more precise measurement can be made under these circumstances. For obvious reasons, however, this technique is seldom done in the laboratory situation and is used primarily in a research setting.

The volume of gas which does remain in the lungs at the end of a maximal forced expiration – the residual volume – is calculated by subtracting the Expiratory Reserve Volume (ERV) from the Functional Residual Capacity

2*

(FRC). The Total Lung Capacity (TLC), the amount of gas remaining in the lung at the end of a voluntary maximal inspiration is arrived at by adding the Functional Residual Capacity (FRC) to the Inspiratory Capacity (IC).

The glottal status during phonation may be estimated by an aerodynamic study called the aerodynamic vocal function test. Theoretically, glottal resistance (F) during phonation can be calculated from the measures of subglottal pressure (P) and air flow rate (F) during phonation. Specifically this may be expressed by the formula $R = \frac{P}{F}$.

The precise measurement of subglottal pressure requires insertion of a needle into the subglottal space or other equally difficult procedures, and is impractical as a routine clinical test. Newer interpolative studies are approaching this area, however, and may prove to be near enough to the specific measurements, to be useful clinically [57].

Measurement of air flow rate per se can and does provide highly informative data on the glottal status – the degree of glottal closure, for instance. This technique employs a pneumotachograph fitted with a mouthpiece to record the air flow rate while the patient is phonating as for example /a/ for as long as possible, at comfortable pitch and intensity. Recording of the data should be done at the moment when the voice is stable, excluding the readings at the initiation of voice, and at the end. If this is done, the total phonation volume divided by the maximum phonation time will also give the mean flow rate. Measurement of maximum phonation time alone is also useful under circumstances when no measurement with instruments is possible, such as during surgery. In the case of a wide glottal gap, as in recurrent nerve paralysis, the air flow rate during phonation is great (F > 200 cc/sec) and can exceed 500 cc/sec when the gap is extremely wide. Changes in the air flow rate resulting from surgery can be a good indication of effectiveness of the surgery.

In a case of high glottal resistance (hyperfunctional voice disorder), a *low* mean flow rate is observed (F < 100 cc/sec). A low vocal velocity index, calculated as a ratio of mean flow rate to vital capacity, gives an indication of an increase in glottal resistance during phonation. The final calculation made will be the ratio of the phonation volume to vital capacity (PV/VC) – the lower the PV/VC ratio, the higher the glottal resistance. When looked at in toto, all of this information gives us both a fairly accurate and fairly specific picture of how the vocal folds act on the air stream, and can be used quickly to gauge vocal fold approximation, tension, etc.

What do these particular determinants mean and what importance do they have relative either to singing or to speech phonation? Certainly in an asthmatic bronchitis, in an emphysema, where scar tissue impairs mobility of the bronchial and bronchiolar lumens with respiration, and in other irritative and inflammatory states, all of these functions or certain of them may be reduced. It has been surprising to the authors to see how many premiere level operatic singers, for example, when asked to sing in an office practice situation, do demonstrate some sort of allergic or inflammatory impairment of bronchial, bronchiolar or pulmonary function. It is likewise somewhat surprising to see how many of these same individuals do present with some form of asthma, and in turn, with some form of constriction or restriction of their gaseous outflow from the chest.

The busy practitioner will not always have access to this elaborate equipment in his office, or he may not have time to employ if it is available to him. A convenient method of assessing some of these functions in a less accurate, but in a more convenient and immediate way involves asking the subject to take a maximal inspiration and count as many numbers as he can during the expiratory phase. While crude, this does, nonetheless give some idea as to general pulmonary function. In addition, some parameters of phonatory efficiency (which is, of course, the end product with which all of us are primarily concerned) can be arrived at by asking the subject to phonate on expiration with an "s" sound (which is made only by the tongue against the back of the top teeth). The resultant sibilant exhalation time can be measured with the second hand on a watch. If this is then compared with a similar timing of a "z" sound, a measurement of phonatory efficiency will result since the "s" measures the amount of available air which the subject has used. In an ideal circumstance, or at least in a healthy one, the phonated "z" sound should be near the non-phonated "s" sound. If there is a variance, then of course phonatory efficiency is impeded and should be evaluated in more detail at a later time.

3. Acoustic Analyses

Because the ear is a monitor of vocal quality and provides a person with feedback as to the nature of his voice, vocal dynamics testing also includes an acoustic analysis. A recording is made of the patient's voice as he sits in a sound-free booth and phonates several vowels and pitch changes. The tape is then analyzed using a sonograph which gives a time vs. frequency graph of 2.4 seconds of information. The frequency spectrum displayed is 80–8000 Hertz so that the fundamental frequency and most of its harmonics is easily graphed. The speaking pitch level, the fundamental frequency, is easily determined from the sonograph of the vowel /a/. The sonographs of the vowels /a/ and /c/ are then further studied and typed if noise components are present. The harmonic components appear on the sonogram (narrow band filter) as parallel horizontal lines when the vocal pitch is kept constant. The pitch level, or the fundamental frequency to be exact, can be estimated by measuring the frequency interval between these lines [58].

When the voice is hoarse, these horizontal lines, corresponding to harmonics, become vague and instead, an irregular, dotted pattern like a cloud appears rather than the "cleaner" horizontal bands, and this picture delineates the presence of noise components.

The degree of hoarseness can be assessed by determining the ratio of the harmonics (horizontal lines) to noise (cloudy pattern). A changing ratio over repeated testing sessions would be quite significant.

Specific insights into some of these component parts of the respiratory tract physiologic functionings can be very helpful to the patient if one is attempting

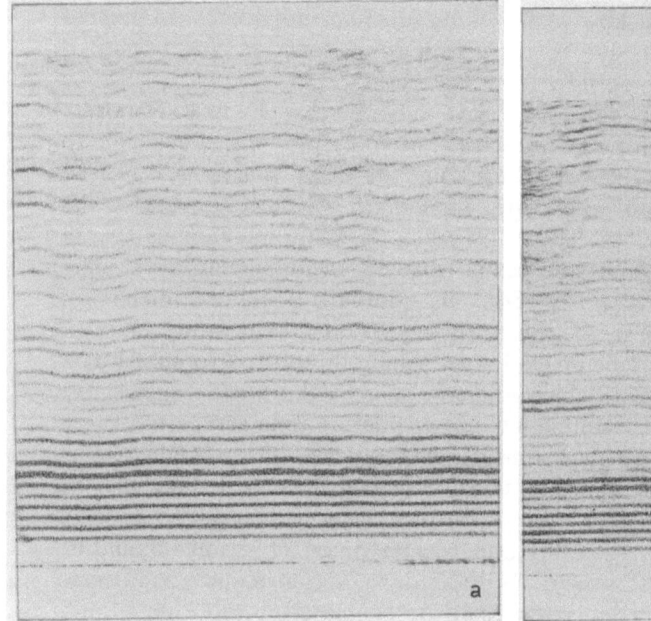
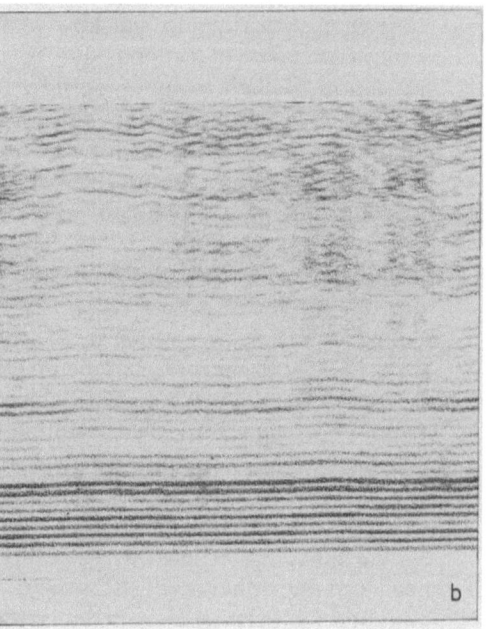
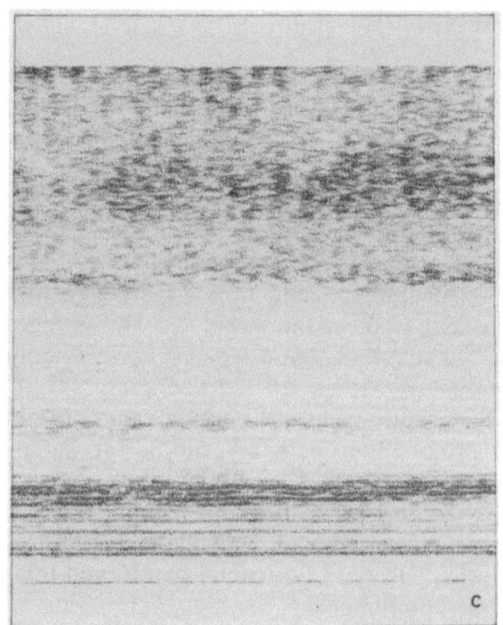

Figs. 4 a–c. Typical examples of sound spectrograms or sonograms: *a* a "normal" sounding voice, *b* and *c* voices with increasingly large noise components in the tracings. Examples *b* and *c* are from patients with a mild viral laryngitis, and a severe laryngo-tracheitis to spotlight or highlight areas where improvement in function is indicated. The ultimate goal of all of us who are concerned with patients in these areas is, of course, that the patient develop an adequate means and an accurate means for automonitoring his voice. Without this, of course, surgery can often be pointless as for example, the removal of a pair of vocal cord nodules in a patient who has failed to develop auditory insight into what his optimum phonatory signal is like. Under these circumstances, it is very possible that the individual will redevelop nodules. It is essential in the successful management of patients with phonatory difficulties that these patients do acquire skills in monitoring themselves adequately and functionally (see Fig. 4).

4. Electrolaryngography

In 1981 at the tenth Symposium on Care of the Professional Voice, a relatively new instrument was introduced in the United States [45]. Its applications were more elaborately ennumerated and described at the 1982 Symposium. This apparatus, called an electroglottograph, has been investigated extensively in the United Kingdom by Adrian Fourcin [43]. The apparatus is an ingenious one and consists of a transmitter of high frequency energy waves or vibrations which are passed from one side of the patient's (lateral) neck, through the soft tissues of the neck and larynx, and then received by a receiver on the contralateral side of the neck. The manufacture of the apparatus is such that with the glottis in a closed position, more energy is transmitted. With the glottis opened, less is received by the receptor attachment. If this energy pattern is then displayed on an oscilloscope screen, the series of wave forms can be described. These correspond very closely to the opened and closed phases of phonation. They may be measured and photographed, and, in addition, the wave form on the oscilloscope screen can be used as a form of teaching device and for biofeedback. The primary use in this context has been by Reed [44], a voice teacher in New York, who feels that crispness of closure pattern on the oscilloscope screen represents efficiency of glottal closure, since optimum voice production depends upon a relatively long closed phase and a relatively short open phase. Heightening the efficiency and production of glottal closure is perceived to strengthen the emitted phonation. By asking his students to "clean up" the clarity of their glottal closure pattern· as indicated on the oscilloscope screen, Reed has found a demonstrable improvement in the crispness and in the clarity of the emitted phonatory signal. Fourcin has also commented and demonstrated that any circumstance which interferes with the efficiency of glottal closure will have a corresponding curve display on the oscilloscope screen. While the electroglottograph is, admittedly, a new instrument, and while its precise applications are not yet entirely clear, it does appear to be a prospectively valuable addition to the armamentarium with which a subject's laryngeal function can be both evaluated and recorded. The recording, incidentally, of the oscilloscope display is made by a Polaroid® camera photograph of the wave form when this is averaged and held constant on the oscilloscope display tube (see Figs. 5 and 6).

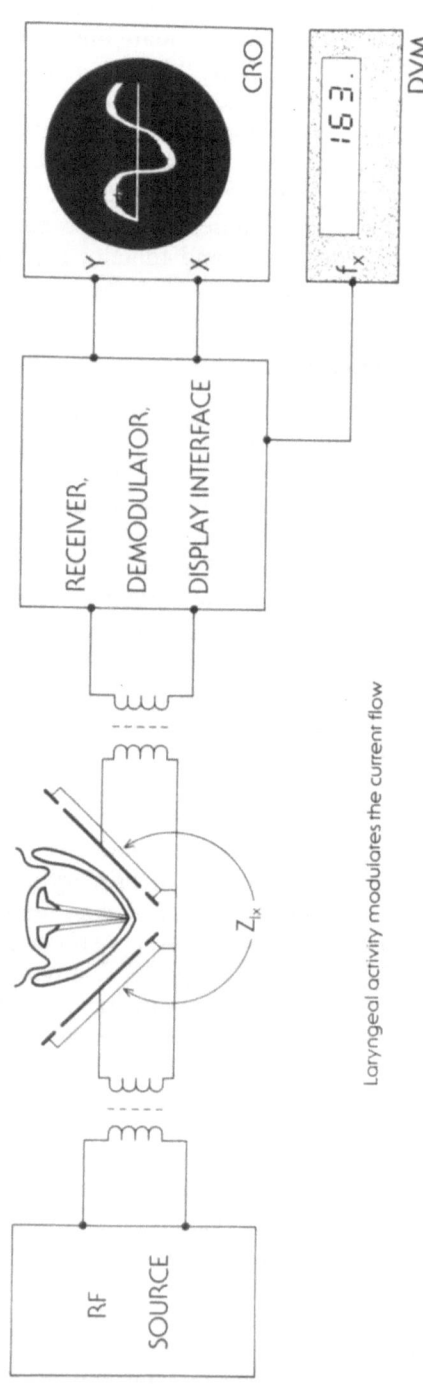

A radio frequency (RF) current is passed through the larynx between two electrodes on either side of the midline of the neck

The current flow is detected by the RF receiver and the variations are demodulated as in AM radio reception

Laryngeal activity modulates the current flow

Figs. 5 and 6. Electroglottograph (electrolaryngograph) tracing and wave form

Fig. 5. The wave form pattern is shown on a cathode ray oscilloscope (CRO) and the frequency (Hertz) of the voice fundamental appears on a digital voice meter (DVM). (Figure taken from: The Electrolaryngograph as a Clinical Tool for the Observation and Analysis of Vocal Fold Vibration, a 1980 exhibit presented jointly in Anaheim, California, by the AAO committee on Laryngeal and Voice Physiology, and the Voice Foundation)

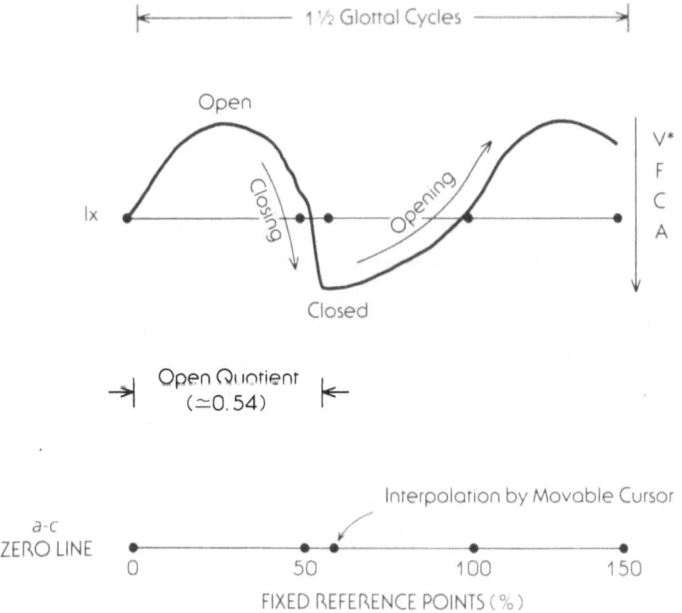

Fig. 6. Wave form display, electrolaryngogram. (Figure taken from: The Electrolaryngograph as a Clinical Tool for Observation and Analysis of Vocal Fold Vibration, a 1980 exhibit presented jointly in Anaheim, California, by the AAO Committee on Laryngeal and Voice Physiology, and the Voice Foundation)

5. Auditory Evaluation of Hoarseness

Auditory evaluation of the hoarse voice is also useful in grading and classifying the hoarseness, and requires only the attentive ear of the examiner.

Subjectively, we often use a 4 point scale: 0 none, 1 slight, 2 fair, 3 extreme. The hoarse voice should also subjectively be judged against the factors of R (rough), B (breathy), A (asthenic) and D (degree) [59].

If we employ such a system, subjectively rating a patient's voice only with the laboratory instrument which is our own (hopefully) trained ear, for example, an "R" type hoarseness suggests a laryngeal polyp and "RB" could suggest laryngeal cancer. The notation of this sort of evaluation and conclusion on the patient record will be quite valuable for another examiner and also, exceedingly cost-effective. Whether or not there is any question that a hearing problem may be related to the vocal complaint, auditory tests should also be performed. The duration of a hearing loss must be ascertained. A temporary condition may result in different vocal problems from those which occur when hearing is permanently impaired. A choral singer who attempts to match his perceived loudness level against that of his peers and who has permanent sensorineural losses may have far-ranging vocal difficulties.

A thorough evaluation of a patient by these methods can thus provide a fairly detailed, and fairly accurate evaluation of respiratory tract physiologic functionings, and thereby, invaluable insight into his vocal problems.

6. X-Ray Studies

As another *general diagnostic* tool, radiologic methods provide a further approach for diagnosis. Soft tissue X-rays of the neck and the larynx, for instance, may be taken in order to show gross vocal fold contours, a subglottic stenosis, or the position and appearance of the false cords when these are seen in the PA view. The lateral film can be especially helpful to show the epiglottis, the cricoid, and its posterior aspect in relationship to the posterior hypopharyngeal wall, and in answering the very common concern in mirror-laryngoscopy (discussed later) as to whether any of these structures is displaced.

7. Tomography

Tomography, or sectional roentgenography, is another X-ray technique to demonstrate, layer by layer, the inter-relationships between structures at different depths of the tissues being examined [60]. Tomography is usually done with the X-ray beam focused in depth increments of 0.5 cm, but other depth definitions are possible. Tomography is the technique of choice in outlining the physical form of the vocal folds, primarily in the PA view. Though rarely used, lateral views may also be made. This sectional analysis can demonstrate, in more detail than conventional X-ray, the different depths of the larynx, and is, therefore, useful to show the vocal folds and the ventricular bands, their relative position during phonation and respiration, and whether or not a paralysis or subglottic stenosis is present. (When one vocal fold is paralyzed, the involved fold is sometimes lower than the intact one, and this has important implications in treatment.) The trachea can also be examined by tomography, again usually in a PA view. The film shows the gross position of the trachea and can also delineate some small deviations of the lateral wall.

The technique of tomography is an ingenious one and its successful accomplishment depends upon moving the film as well as the X-ray tube with respect to the patient during a particular exposure. Specifically, both are moved around a center point which has been calculated to fall in the plane of the area which is to be studied and if this is done, the structures which are not in the plane selected for study will appear to be blurred and intentionally so since they will be moving relative to the film itself. A quick investigation of the diagram (Fig. 7) shows if one is studying the larynx (1), it will appear in sharp detail on the film while the shadow of an object at (2) will be magnified, blurred and distorted to lie between points A and B on the film. Only those laryngeal structures which are in the plane of the pivot point will appear in sharp focus, and the blurred outline lacking detail, which represents anatomy which lies either behind or in front of the larynx, will be distorted in such a way that no recognizable image will appear. This resultant "soft focus" or blurring will be such that the eye easily can ignore it.

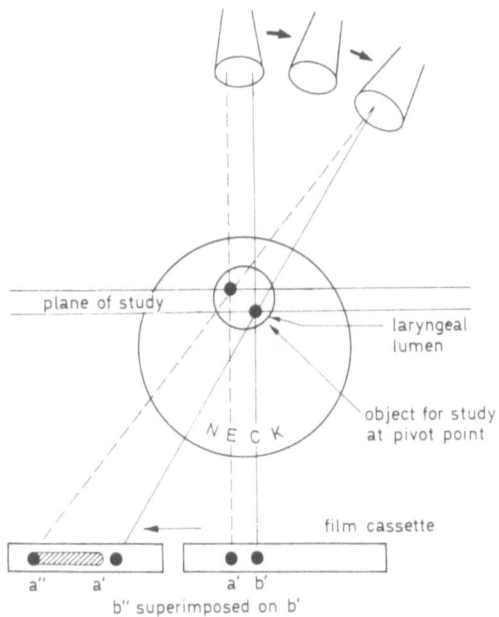

plane of study

laryngeal lumen

object for study at pivot point

N E C K

film cassette

a″   a′   a′ b′
b″ superimposed on b′

TOMOGRAM FOR A CORONAL SLICE

Fig. 7. Schematic diagrammatic schema for tomography.
(Redrawn from Squires, L: Fundamentals of Radiology. Cambridge: Harvard Univ. Press. 1982)

8. Computerized Axial Tomography

This is a very provocative new radiologic examination procedure which is currently assuming an increasing prominence, and is used for study of all body parts and of the larynx as well. This is an X-ray procedure which was first developed in England and which was given its first practical clinical application in 1973. Its unique contribution to the diagnostic armamentarium lies in the fact that by computer-aiding the X-ray images which are obtained by relatively conventional tomographic techniques, increasingly small differences in density of the tissues in question can be visualized. This computer-enhancement has been of its greatest value, perhaps, in visualizing the brain, but it has an equally valid and an equally exciting application in visualization of the larynx.

In one of the more usual configurations or CT Scanner design (Fig. 8), both the X-ray emitting source and the X-ray detector source rotate continually in a 180° arc about the patient. The electronic detector receives the tissue-transmitted information and amplifies it as electrical pulses which are then recorded and stored for computer reference. These impulses, of course, will vary, just as they do on the X-ray film according to the density or lack of

density of the medium through which they are passing. The electronic
detection device is approximately 100 times more sensitive to the gradations in
X-ray beam (and thereby, to the gradation in absorption of X-ray beam by
tissues) than is conventional X-ray film.

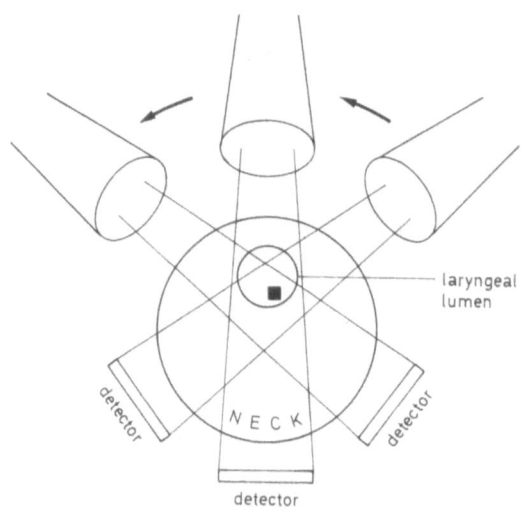

COMPUTERIZED TOMOGRAPHY

Fig. 8. Diagrammatic schema for computerized tomography.
(Redrawn from Squires, L: Fundamentals of Radiology. Cambridge: Harvard Univ. Press. 1982)

If a portion of the anatomy being considered contains more inorganic
calcium (or other metal) than the tissue surrounding it does, a greater part of
the X-ray beam passing through that area will be absorbed or attenuated each
time it is recorded by the electronic detector and by its affiliated computer.
The tissue substance which is not so dense and in the vicinity will absorb
relatively little of the radiographic energy by comparison and the detector, in
turn, will record a higher intensity of X-ray beam as it, in turn, records and
reports to the computer.

An averaging is then done by the computer for each of the component
areas which make up the X-ray "slice" and among this tissue will be, for
example, a portion of a cervical vertebra. The resulting computer number
averages are then printed on a computer paper readout, and this, in turn,
would represent numerically the component density of all of the tissue
substrata which lie in the area of study. The numerical values which the
computer produces represents the density of the tissue substrate of the slice
from which the readings are taken. Areas of high density are surrounded by
areas of less density. The density numbers which are printed by the computer,
incidentally, relate to the absorption values of the small areas of tissue which
they represent in contrast to that of water. Water is arbitrarily given a value of

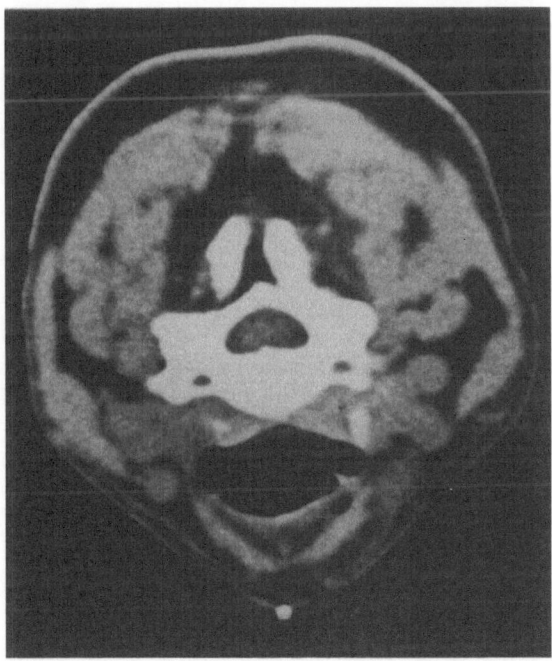

Fig. 9a. The dense osseous structure of the cervical vertebra is well shown. The cavity of the hypopharynx anterior to it is delineated and on the left of the picture, the sternomastoid muscle is particularly well defined

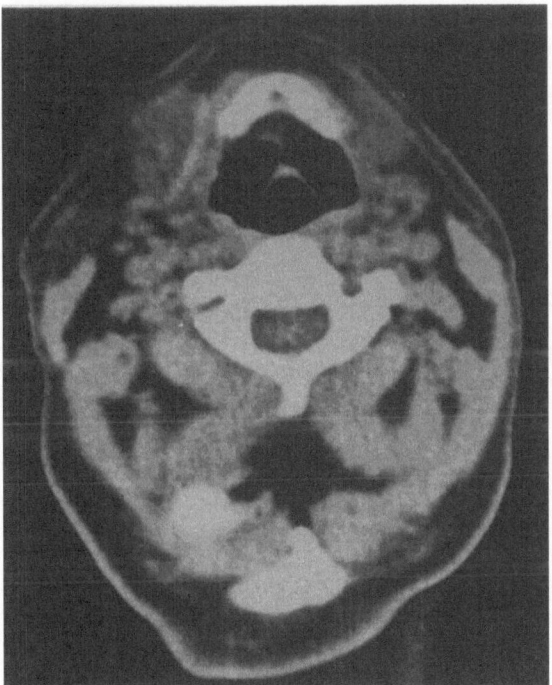

Fig. 9b. Within the air-containing space of the hypopharynx can be seen the very tip of the epiglottis. Almost touching it is the hyoepiglottic ligament anteriorly continuing toward the hyoid bone. The hyoid in this patient appears to have been pierced by the thyroglossal duct in its migration inferiorly in the neck

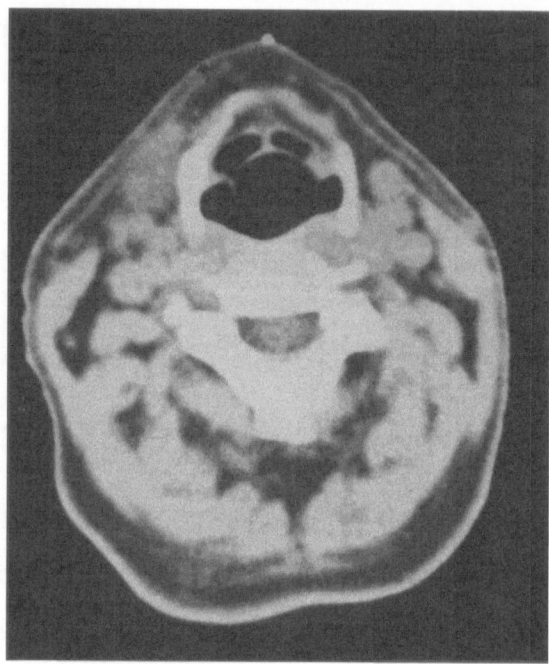

Fig. 9c. The inferior cornu of the hyoid bone is seen at the lateral extension of the ovoid hypopharynx. The glossoepiglottic ligament is well defined extending anteriorly and is flanked by the lobed vallecula on either side

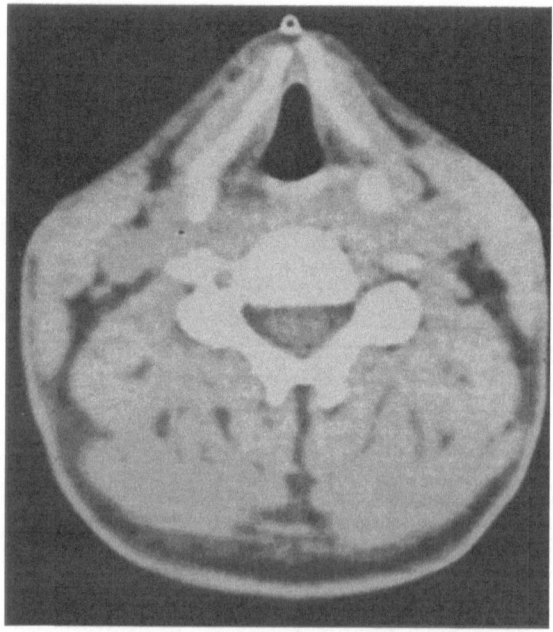

Fig. 9d. The two thyroid cartilage lamina have not yet fused anteriorly to produce the thyroid prominence on the anterior neck. The bulge within the air space probably represents the beginning of the vestibular fold on either side. Inferiorly and on the right side, the superior cornu of the thyroid cartilage is seen as a discrete circular entity

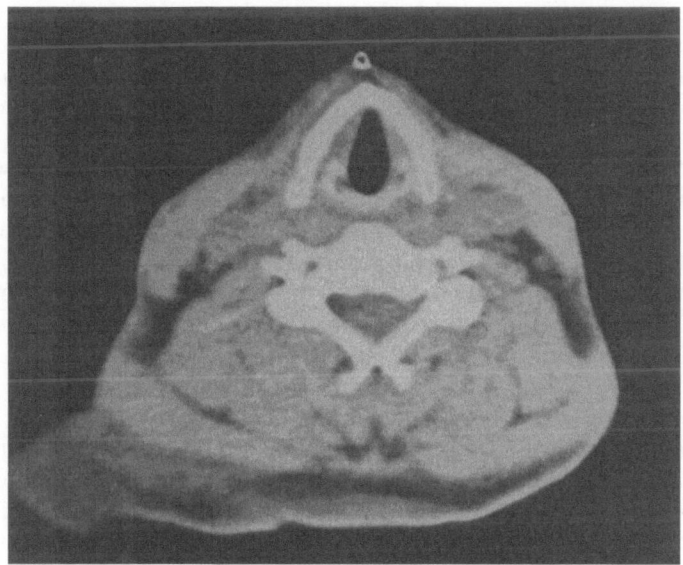

Fig. 9e. Within the firmly conjoined thyroid lamina of the two sides, the interior of the larynx is now visible. A small portion of the arytenoid cartilage is seen near the posterior end of the air space and the upper portion of the signet-ring-shaped crycoid cartilage begins to appear. This particular scan marks the approximate level of the true vocal fold

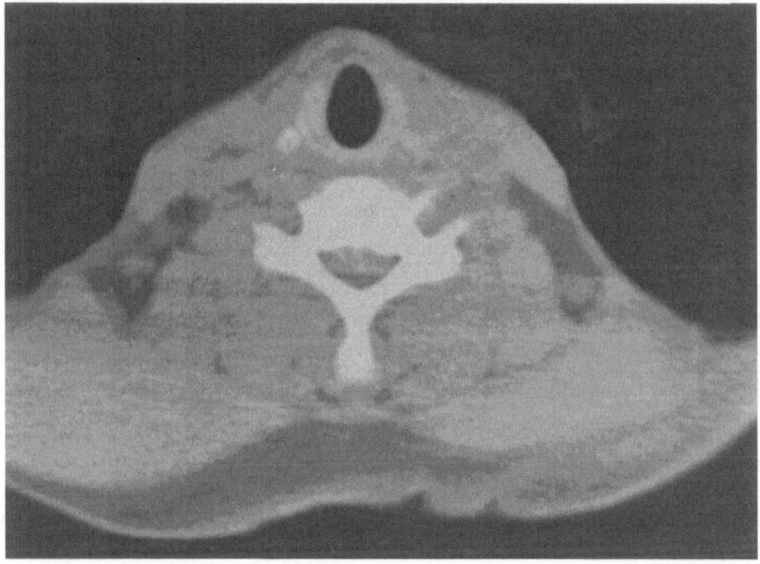

Fig. 9f. The ovoid-shaped subglottal air space is well defined. The inferior cornu of the thyroid cartilage is particularly well defined on the left of the photograph. The crycoid cartilage shows relatively little calcification on this particular view

zero. Materials, or tissues, which then have absorption values greater than water (as for example bone or cartilage) will have a CT computer number which will be a positive one (this is expressed in Houndsfield units, after one of the inventors of the CT technique). Tissues which have densities less than water will be expressed as negative numbers. For example air is -500 and bone is given a value of $+500$. Muscle, cartilage and blood, for example, would all lie somewhere in between those numbers. These density numbers are then given a specific shade of black or gray or white and will be viewed almost immediately on a television screen monitor.

This image will then come to indicate the radiographic density (or lack of density) of the slice of body tissue being studied. Since as mentioned earlier, this technique involves electronics approximately 100 times more sensitive than conventional X-ray film, it can provide us with a much more accurate configuration of the tissue areas studied than all antecedent methods. It is, as a consequence, quite easy to understand why Computerized Axial Tomography or "Cat Scans" (CAT, CT, CTT, EMI – all are synonymous) has rapidly taken a front position in regards to the question of radiographic diagnosis of soft tissue structures. Permanent images, incidentally, which have been obtained by photographing such a television monitor screen are shown in Fig. 9a–f showing "sclices" of computer aided tomographic views of a normal larynx.

9. Laryngogram

Another X-ray technique is the laryngogram, which relies upon the use of a contrast medium to outline the walls of the mucosal surface of the larynx. Usually this contrast medium will be an oily substance containing a radio-opaque material such as iodine. It is performed and photographed with fixed film X-rays, motion pictures or TV film. Tissue movements are observed in fluoroscopy and still pictures can be taken at any time during the laryngographic examination.

The velopharyngeal area can also be examined with all of these radiographic techniques. The aim here is usually to detect any nasopharyngeal mass or obstruction to closure and to assess the available nasopharyngeal space. Velopharyngeal closure in vowel production during speech is well demonstrated during cine-fluorography, for example. The cross sectional area of the velopharynx can be measured by using computed tomography (CT) scanning.

10. Xeroradiography

A final radiographic technique used in physical diagnosis and evaluation of the larynx and of the entire neck is that of xeroradiography. This technique utilizes a specially coated metal plate which is developed after exposure, without the use of liquid chemicals. The metal plate in turn is composed of a metal base coated with a layer of semi-conductor material, usually a form of selenium. This material has the capacity of retaining an electrical charge while in the

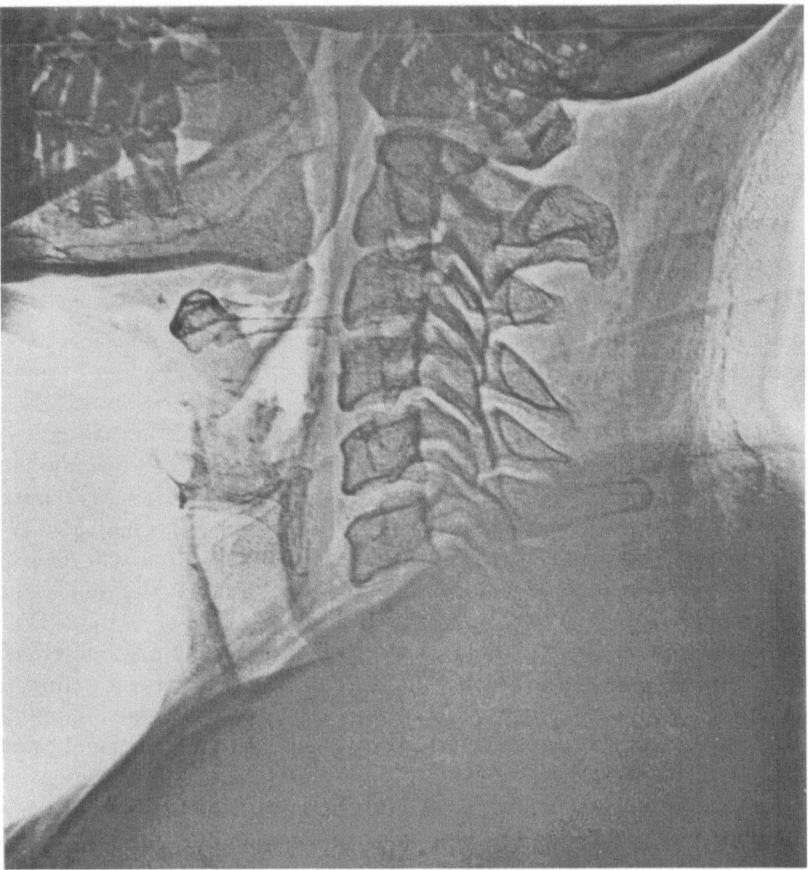

Fig. 10. Lateral xerogram of normal larynx. Beneath the relatively horizontal line made by the lower edge of the mandible can be seen the similarly horizontal hyoid bone. Within its two cornu can be seen the epiglottis which just appears to touch against the angle of the mandible. Below the epiglottis is the shield-shaped thyroid cartilage with a relatively small thyroid prominence (this is probably a female patient) and below the thyroid cartilage the vague outline of the signet-ring-shaped cryoid cartilage can be seen. There is a small discrete accessory immediately inferior to the one cornu of the hyoid bone. These triticeous cartilages appear on an estimated 26% of xeroradiograms

dark (it is dissipated by exposure to visible light). The metal base plate is charged in a special chamber from a high voltage direct current source. The metal plate is then exposed to X-rays in the usual way. The plate is then developed (dry) in a dark room which is a specially prepared chamber. When the surface plate is dusted with powder, the powder will be taken up by the surface of the plate in proportion to the electrical charge which the plate retains. In this way an image is outlined. As a consequence of the refraction of the X-ray beams at the edges of different densities and of structures, there is an edge enhancement. As a consequence this technique permits the procedurement of beautiful soft tissue detail which would otherwise be non-visible if a standard X-ray beam with a standard X-ray plate were utilized. This diagnostic technique was felt at its inception to offer much potential, but its position has now been preempted in most institutions by the newer computerized tomography radiographic techniques. Fig. 10 demonstrates a xeroradiograph of a lateral view of the neck.

C. Patient Records

The final paragraph in this chapter relating to history and to physical diagnosis addresses perhaps one of the most important points: the keeping of adequate *patient records*. At the first interview of a patient who presents with a vocal complaint it is extremely important to make a recording of the patient's voice. We all have a miserably inaccurate acoustic memory of how we sound, and of how others sound. Recordings, usually acoustic tapes, serve as a basis for subsequent comparison in several contexts. Once the abnormal quality of a patient's voice is surgically corrected, the patient very often will forget how severe the disorder had been, and well may not realize the full extent of improvement, unless it is demonstrated to him by a tape recording. Both for benefit of the patient and the therapists as well, a recording made after surgery can be compared with the initial one, and then later still with those done subsequent to the post-surgical therapy. Since it is difficult, meaningfully and qualitatively to describe vocal quality, these tapes serve as permanent records. For these reasons, as well as to evaluate the success of treatment, vocal dynamics testing should be performed both before and after therapy. Photographs and TV recordings may also be obtained and retained with the patient's records visually to highlight the acoustic improvements which result from treatment. At the very least, auditory tapes should be made of any patient's voice when the otolaryngic surgeon proposes a surgical procedure aimed at improving voice quality.

Patient Examination via the Endolaryngeal Approach: Diagnosis and Therapy 3

For a complete examination of the nasopharynx, and then the larynx, including the arytenoids, vestibular and true vocal folds, trachea, hypopharyngeal wall, introitus of the esophagus, the anterior commissure, aryepiglottic folds, vallecula, pyriform sinuses, epiglottis and base of the tongue – one of several indirect laryngoscopic techniques may be utilized. The term "indirect laryngoscopy" is used since these structures are viewed indirectly and not with the eyes of the examiner directly inspecting them. Usually, this is done either by the use of a mirror, to reflect the visual image, or by an optical system using reflected light for visual transmission to obtain an image. In addition to using it for diagnostic procedures, some laryngologists use indirect laryngoscopy to assist in the performance of surgical procedures (Fig. 12).

Mirror laryngoscopy is the simplest form of indirect visualization and follows a technique popularized by Manuel Garcia, a singing teacher, over a hundred years ago.

The history of indirect laryngoscopy is a lengthy and interesting one and we owe to Manuel Garcia (1805–1906) [35] our first real concern with a view of the living, functioning larynx. Previous to Garcia, many medical researchers and many medical authors had conjectured about voice and sometimes with surprising accuracy considering the strictures which prevailed for so many years with respect to dissection of the human body.

It would appear that Hippocrates probably was aware that sound originated in the chest. Later, Aristotle philosophized that voice was related anatomically in some way to heart and soul. The founding father, however, of the science of laryngology was Claudius Galen [46].

It would appear that Galen enjoyed the reverence of his peers and also of his ruler, for he served as personal physician to the Roman Emperor, Marcus Aurelius, and on at least one occasion, was brought back from his travels to Rome when his attention was demanded by the Emperor. Galen seems to have been the first "physician", in the sense that we know them, to have based his

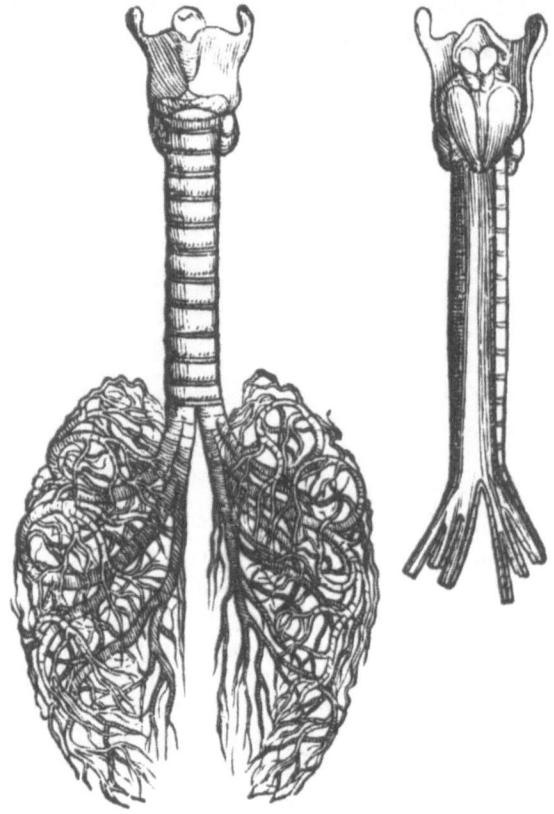

Fig. 11. Tracheobronchial tree.
(Woodcut from Vesalius' De Humani Corporis Fabrica; 1542 A.D.)

concept of physiology and his awareness of anatomy on personal observations. These were made both apparently on cadaver specimens and on animal specimens as well. Those physicians and those authors who followed Galen over the next 1,500 years did very little to advance our knowledge either of the anatomy or of the physiology of larnygeal function and the maxims which Galen had laid down in the first century of the Christian era remained virtually unchallenged or unquestioned through the Renaissance.

Interestingly enough, it is to a very famous artist, Leonardo da Vinci (1452–1519) to whom we owe our next anatomically detailed drawings of the larynx and of the laryngeal structures, and an example of his principal effort in this matter, Quarderni d'Anatomia [36] was published circa 1500. Leonardo clearly seems to have understood both the anatomy, form and function of the larynx as he has indicated it in his sketches of the larynx and also seems to have assigned the importance of the mouth, teeth, lips and tongue for articulation. Regrettably this effort remained undiscovered for approximately 300 years. It is now, however, one of the prize possessions of the British Royal Family. Interest in the specific formation of phonated sound, however, appears to have been accomplished by a French physician, Antonie Ferrein [37] (1693–1769) and he appears to have been the first scholar to use the excised cadaver larynx for acoustic production. It seems to have been Ferrein who first discribed the similarity between vocal fold movement and movement of vibrating strings, least so far as the relation between length and pitch is concerned. It is he who termed the vibratory edges forming the rima glottidis "vocal cords" which is a term still used today.

In 1542, Andreas Vesalius [47] published his monumental atlas of anatomy, De Humani Corporis Fabrica. Composed of a series of beautifully executed woodents (see Fig. 11) and with some attributed to the then contemporary artist Titian, this work demonstrated how far the knowledge of anatomy of the larynx and bronchial tree had progressed by that time.

On March 13, 1855, Manuel Garcia (1805–1906) as noted earlier, a prominent teacher of singing was in London, and presented his observations "Physiological Observations on the Human Voice" to the Royal Academy of Medicine. Garcia seems to have been the first individual to record his observations on his own larynx and this feat was accomplished with the use of a small dental mirror and with sunlight reflected from a mirror held in his other hand. In this way, he was able to view his own larynx in action, and is the person to whom we credit mirror laryngoscopy. He attempted to use this as a basis for teaching his students of voice through his teaching career. The reader, incidentally, who is interested in more detail than is given here should see the article by Hans von Leden [34] for more detail. von Leden has made an extensive search of the literature relating to the history of laryngology and has presented it in a more elaborate form in an as yet unpublished address given in 1982 at the Juilliard Symposium on Care of the Professional Voice.

A. Mirror Laryngoscopy

Mirror laryngoscopy or indirect laryngoscopy remains the cornerstone of the clinical practice of laryngology, and has been so since Garcia's popularization/publication of the technique. In this technique, a handled small plane or magnifying mirror is used to reflect the laryngeal area. The exact size of mirror, and its reflective qualities selected by the examiner should be initially, the largest in size that can be used comfortably in the pharynx of a particular patient. Fogging of the mirror can be prevented by several means, and usually is accomplished by warming the glass by any one of several means. Before introducing the mirror into the patient's oropharynx, the examiner is admonished to reassure the patient, to instruct him how to breathe, and to warn him not to be concerned if he gags. Individual response varies considerably. A trained singer can usually demonstrate the larynx quite adequately. In other patients, however, a local anesthetic, such as 2% pontocaine or 4% xylocaine, may be applied. (Details on anesthesia will be discussed in a later section). The position taken by the patient depends upon the examining instrumentation, and upon the preferences of the examiner. It is preferable to have the patient sit up straight, with his neck and head projected slightly forward. The examiner sits in front of the patient with his head at the same level as the patient's. Using a piece of gauze to prevent slipping, the examiner grasps the patient's tongue, opposing thumb on the bottom with index finger on top. The third finger is used holding the upper lip away and superior. This provides some advantage over the traditional teaching of holding the thumb on top of the tongue, because it permits that the third finger alternately could be used to help depress the tongue if necessary. With

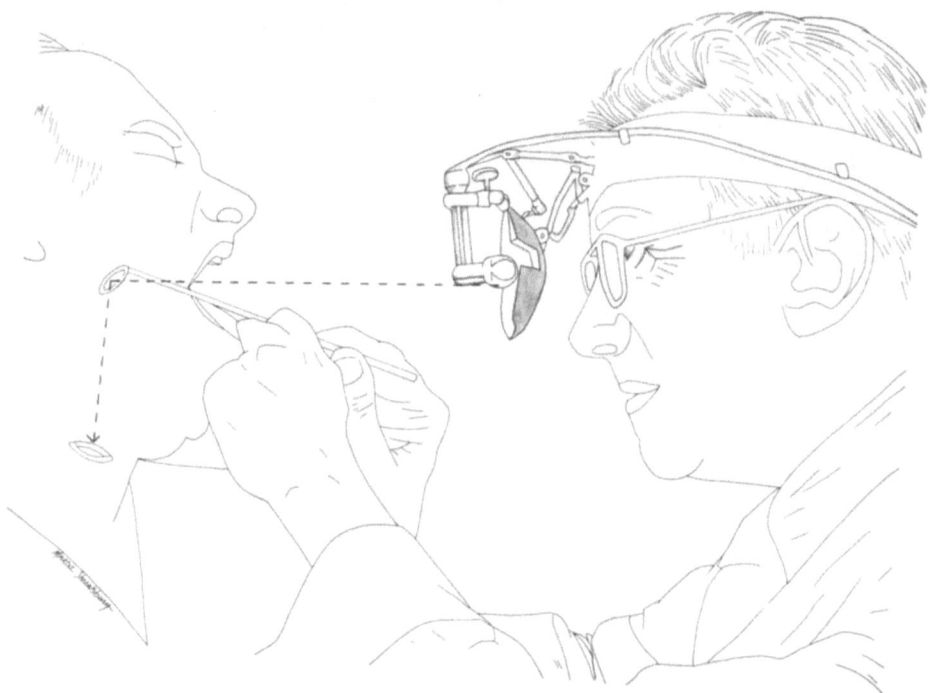

Fig. 12. Indirect (or mirror) laryngoscopy, technique

his illumination source positioned correctly and with light coming from an electric bulb used with head mirror, or any type of self-contained headlight, the examiner gently inserts the laryngeal mirror to the depth of the oropharynx, over the tongue base. Care is taken not to create a sudden motion which could cause gagging. Reassurance, relaxation, and proper breathing must be stressed as the patient is instructed to pant and phonate the /i/ vowel.

The muscular effort associated with the patient's attempt to phonate /i/ in this position brings the larynx up and back and moves the epiglottis forward, permitting a better view of the larynx. Often particularly if the patient is a singer, the examiner may request that the patient go through an entire scale while the tongue is held, thereby permitting observation of the larynx in motion and at the extremes of the pitch range. The examiner also may need to keep the mirror in motion, tilting it this way and that for a better view, changing its angle with the long axis of the hypopharynx and larynx as the tract adjusts for changes in pitch.

Vocal fold mobility can grossly be estimated by asking the patient to cough. Cough can also be utilized for clearing the throat when mucus adheres to the edge of the vocal fold, primarily at the junction of the anterior and middle thirds, and often may appear to mimic a more serious problem to the less-experienced examiner.

Mirror laryngoscopy can also be used in conjunction with a Zeiss microscope or its equivalent, employing either the microscope's normal light or a stroboscopic light source. Stroboscopic illumination is useful at times because it facilitates visualization of small lesions which vibrate at variable speeds, out of synchrony with the remainder of the laryngeal structure. The larynx vibrational patterns are not invariable and symmetrical ones, however, even in the same subject. Microscopic mirror laryngoscopy can be of exceeding value to outline the extent of a discoloration, to clarify the examiner's impression of the surface appearance of a vocal fold or a lesion there (and this has many clinical ramifications), of the vibratile edge of the fold (is it really regular and smooth or not?) and of the appearance of the vascular structures which are visible: are they tortuous or are they strongly linear? These, too, have clinical significance. Finally, is there a lack of mucosal surface continuity? This may be a deciding factor in permitting vocal performance in the immediate future.

B. Fiberoptic Laryngoscopy

Fixed fiberoptic laryngoscopy, another indirect visualization technique, employs a rigid fiberoptically lighted device. These instruments can employ no magnification, or can go up to magnification of about 3X. Such a device is used much in the same manner as one utilizes a tongue depressor. The Gould laryngoscope, one such device, presents the following features: 1) "Cold" light at the viewing head is supplied by fiberoptic bundles from an outside source, furnishing ample illumination of the entire viewing field. Lighting is sufficient for good direct visualization and as well for various types of photography, including high-speed cinematography. 2) There is uniform 2.7 magnification of the entire viewing field so that minor lesions may readily be visualized. 3) The laryngoscope requires no traction on the patient's tongue once inserted and, therefore, is often intrinsically more comfortable than conventional instruments; a more "relaxed" and hence more productive laryngoscopic examination is likely (see Figs. 13 and 14). These instruments require skill and dexterity on the part of the examiner, and gentleness as well, but they are far more accessible to the neophyte laryngoscopist than is the effective use of the laryngeal mirror, particularly when the mirror is used, as it often is, with a reflective mirror headlight source on the examiner's head, whose movements and positions must also be coordinated with those of the patient's hypopharynx, oropharynx and larynx.

Flexible fiberoptic laryngoscopy, as its name implies, utilizes a flexible, fiberoptically lighted instrument for visualization of the larynx and

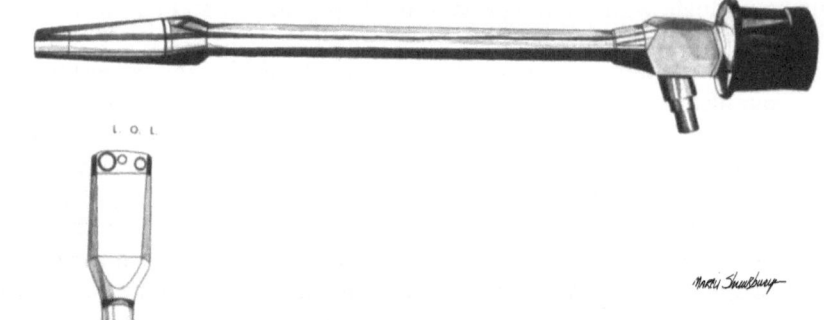

Fig. 13. Rigid fiberoptic (Gould) laryngoscope

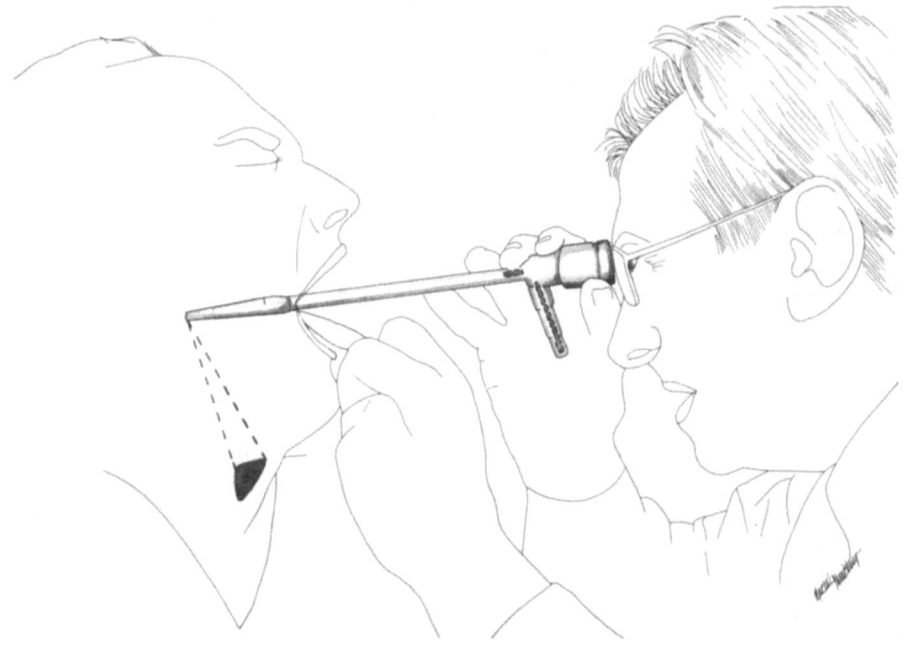

Fig. 14. Gould laryngoscope: technique of use

nasopharynx. Since it is introduced through the nose, an evaluation of the nasal airway for patency sufficient to permit passage of the instrument must be performed to determine which side is spatially more adequate for the procedure. A local anesthetic, such as xylocaine or cocaine, is then customarily applied nasally to permit easier instrumental introduction. Topical anesthesia of the nose and oropharynx is a variable point, however, and the authors differ in choice. The flexible nasopharyngeal-laryngoscope does not have to be heated prior to its introduction, as clearing and cleansing of the lens is effected by the washing of the patient's own mucus during the swallowing act. Its 4 mm diameter and usually 180° tip deflection permit examination of the nasopharynx as the instrument is passed on its way to the larynx. Again, the authors vary in choice here, but two people are usually needed to maneuver the instrument: an assistant will use one hand to hold the viewing laryngoscope for the examiner. The assistant's second hand serves to prevent the instrument from advancing further into the nose, and the examiner then has free use of both his hands. He can then hold the tongue slightly forward to facilitate visualization. He can also perform surgical prodecures with forceps held in either, or possibly instruments held in each hand (see Figs. 15 and 16).

Fiberoptic laryngoscopy also has another value, another dimension which makes it different from virtually all of the other indirect examination techniques. It permits, without the potential hazards of irradiation, observation of virtually all of the structures of the vocal tract, at least from soft palate or oro- and hypopharynx and larynx, as these structures are in use functioning in an almost unimpeded manner. The area from the base of the tongue forward; the mouth, teeth and lips remain out of view to indirect examination. Certainly, it would be inappropriate to expect concert calibre performance of an actor or of a singer who probably has been topically anesthetized and who has a 4 mm, firm but flexible bundle placed in nose, nasopharynx, oropharynx and hypopharynx, but it comes as close to this ideal as has yet been possible of attainment. With mirror, and with the angulated, fixed fiberoptic instruments, the examiner is quite limited and can see little more than /i/ when most subjects phonate. Certainly this has been of enormous value, and still is, and is a basic part of the examination of any larynx. The rigid fiberoptic indirect laryngoscope also has this same limitation, but to a lesser degree. With the flexible instrument, however, the subject can (within limitations) alter head and neck angulations and positions, and can phonate, speak, sing in almost a normal manner. Marginal abnormalities of motion of laryngeal structures other than the vocal folds can be observed, and in running discourse in normal speech, and in singing. When this instrument is coupled with a television camera, and recordings are made as the entire spectrum of laryngeal movements transpire during any given phonatory tasks, permanent records are acquired which will have both diagnostic and prognostic (and legal) significance. Some speech therapists and voice teachers have been quick to perceive the potential value of this instrumentation as a teaching and even as a biofeedback device. Showing a patient or a subject in a hand-held mirror what his tongue or oropharynx looks like, or does in a given situation has always been possible. And with a modicum of dexterity and coordination, a similar demonstration of the endolarynx can be made to the patient/subject of his larynx. But only on /i/, and on scales, at best. With this flexible nasolaryngoscope, plus television camera, plus television recorder and monitor screen, one can easily demonstrate to patient/subject, or to a number of viewers, the endolaryngeal postures and movements during a variety of situations including running speech and artistic level singing performance. The authors are united in their conviction that in this specific combination of instruments a surge in learning and comprehending laryngeal actions, laryngeal physiology in a variety of situations will occur in the coming years.

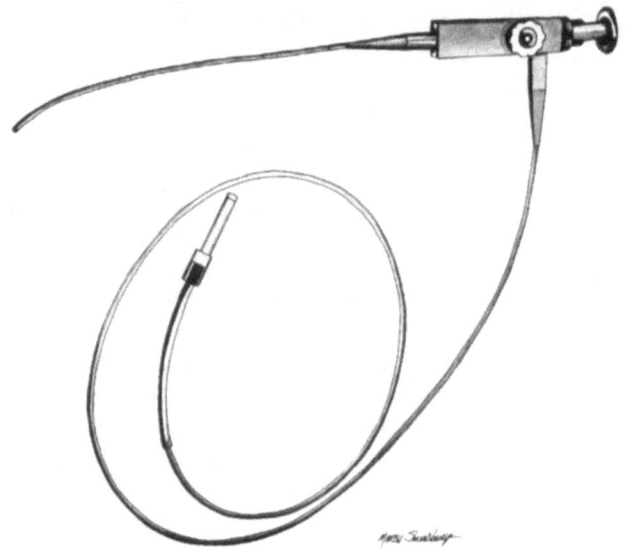

Fig. 15. Flexible fiberoptic laryngoscope

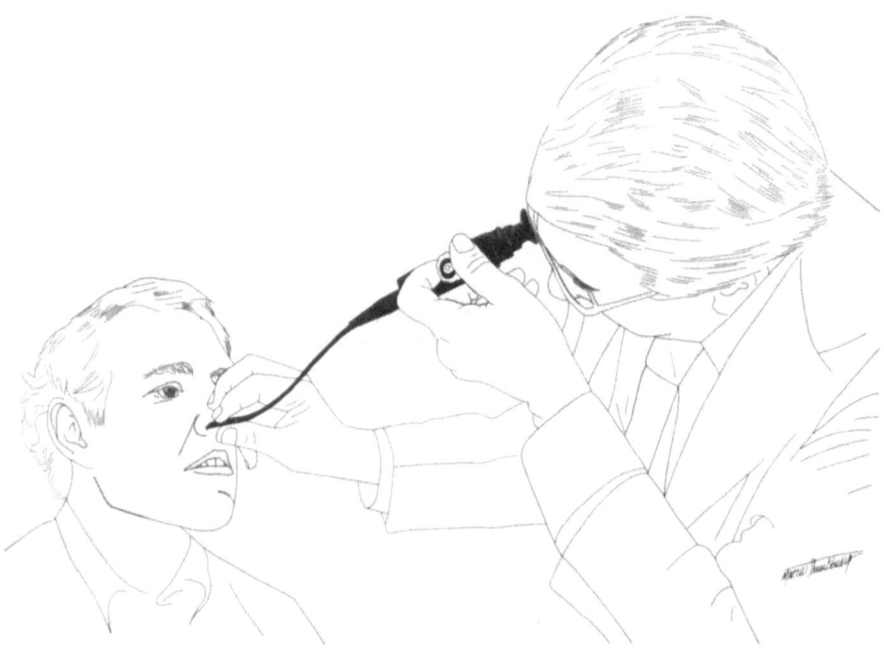

Fig. 16. Flexible fiberoptic laryngoscope; technique of use

C. Indirect Laryngoscopic Surgery

1. Discussion

As earlier mentioned, besides being a diagnostic tool, indirect laryngoscopy can be also used in association with certain *indirect laryngoscopic surgical procedures.* Gross biopsy of lesions is sometimes performed indirectly as, for example, with questionable granulomas, polyps, nodules. With indirect visualization and with a topically anesthetized subject, it is possible to palpate motion of the cricoarytenoid joint and to palpate suspected edema within Reinke's pouch. The advantage of surgery with indirect laryngoscopy is that the surgical procedure can be performed while the patient is awake and subsequent vocal fold alteration changes can immediately be heard.

2. Teflon Injection

Teflon or polytef injections are sometimes used to help paralytic dysphonia or other glottal closure insufficiencies by moving the paralyzed vocal fold closer to the midline so that the functioning fold can meet it and effectively close the glottis. This procedure is specifically facilitated with indirect laryngoscopy, and probably is the method of choice for undertaking this particular surgery. The technique, as described by Dedo, calls for anesthesia of the undersurface of the anterior tongue and the hypopharynx with 2% pontocaine spray [2]. Further local anesthesia is used to obtund the cough reflex. The larynx is visualized in the indirect mirror, as earlier described, and after the application procedure starts, one to three 0.5 cc aliquots of 5% cocaine are dripped on the epiglottis and vocal folds of the patient. Once cough is obtunded, and the larynx thoroughly visualized, the surgeon makes the first injection of the polytef. Customarily this is done, and a Bruening laryngeal syringe is used, injecting into posterolateral corner of the middle third of the vocal fold just anterior to the vocal process, until this section of the fold swells to the midline. A limited time is available for the manipulation, for edema results quickly from the trauma of injection. In certain cases, because of a residual concavity, a second injection may be made in the anterolateral corner of the middle third of the vocal fold just below the edge of the false fold. When the procedure is completed, the glottis is observed indirectly, in the laryngeal mirror. For an optimum result, the injected fold should appear straight, firmly meeting the opposite membranous fold. The quality of phonation should be clear and firm, as opposed to the breathy, weak, and hoarse voice which existed prior to the injection. This should be perceived both by the surgeon and the patient, and recorded acoustically, at the end of the procedure. Care should be taken by the surgeon when he uses teflon to avoid over-injection or injection which is too close to the vocal margin, for any of these maneuvers can cause the fold to be immobilized and become non-vibratile. Injecting too deeply should also be avoided as the teflon may be deposited subglottically and spreading may progress to the thyroarytenoid muscle, affecting its function and thereby

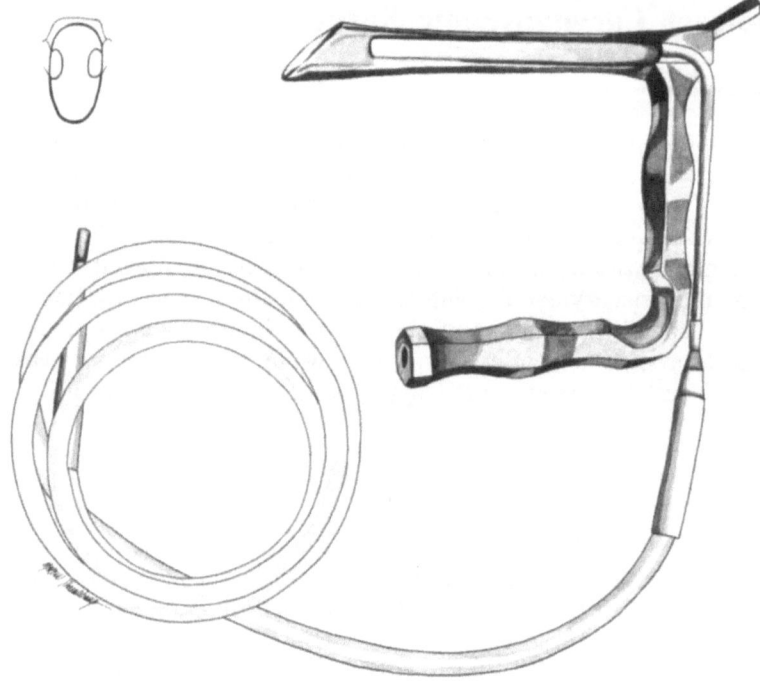

Fig. 17. Anterior commissure (Gould) laryngoscope

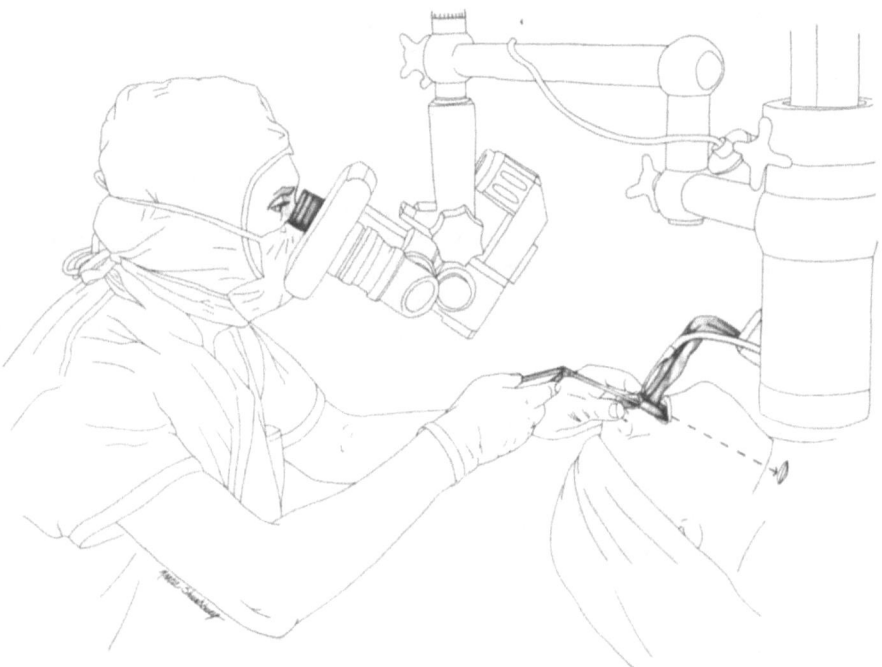

Fig. 18. Direct suspension laryngoscopy. Note use of microscope

causing the voice to be variably weak, breathy, and hoarse [3]. Teflon injections may also be used to assist closure of the velopalatine gap and to reduce chronic, excessive patency of the eustachian tube opening in the torus tubarius area [4]. See "Recommended Reading for Cordal Injection" in References, pp. 109, 110.

D. Direct Laryngoscopy

Direct laryngoscopy is another basic technique in the evaluation of the larynx. Here, the larynx, vocal folds, and adjacent structures are viewed directly by the surgeon as opposed to a view of the reflected images obtained with indirect laryngoscopy. Direct laryngoscopy is now most frequently accomplished with a metal tube or similar device whose distal aperture is illuminated (with incandescent bulb or fiberoptically) and both the light and the viewed image may be intensified with a magnifying apparatus or microscope (see Figs. 17 and 18).

1. Proximal Light Direct Laryngoscopy

This technique, employing a light source proximal to the observer, was first developed by Bruening in 1910 [5]. Because the examining tube does not carry a light source, it is smaller, less complex and more widely open than is its fiberoptically lit counterpart. Several light sources have been utilized, the simplest being a headlight worn by the examiner. The microscope as a light source, an innovation introduced by Kleinsasser, offers one of the best solutions, because, in addition to projecting light, the microscope can permit magnified stereoscopic visualization [6]. Robert has taken advantage of this principle and added a Prades' light deflecting shield to eliminate reflection of the microscope light from the edge of the laryngoscope. In addition, he has vertically narrowed and laterally enlarged the proximal opening to facilitate introduction of the instrument into all but the smallest larynges yet still permit stereoscopic visualization of the interior.

2. Suspension Laryngoscopy

"The Gallows", a direct laryngoscopic suspension examining device designed by Killian in 1910, is another proximally lighted, direct laryngoscope [7]. This apparatus employs an adjustable tongue elevator blade, available in various widths and lengths and connected to a regulating device. That device is, in turn, suspended from an adjustable frame, itself mounted on an operating room table. As the apparatus is cranked upward, pressure is exerted against the tongue blade, pushing the tongue away from the posterior pharyngeal wall. Properly adjusted in all its parts, this instrument produces a broad, stable viewing field. With the assistance of an electric light, it permits wide direct visualization, and easily allows the performance of bimanual manipulation and surgical procedures. When "the gallows" is used, the patient is recumbent and is anesthetized both locally as well as with a general anesthetic. In the hands of a skilled and experienced surgeon, a high degree of precision and facility of use can be obtained from what would sound like a rather ponderous and cumbersome apparatus.

But topical anesthesia cannot be applied to the endolarynx and trachea when an endotracheal tube is in place. Also, the posterior portion of the laryngoscope is open and there is nothing to restrain the endotracheal tube from falling downward and into the operative field which it often does with annoying frequency. This then precludes the use of the modern anesthetic agents which allow for long-term oxygenation and for laryngeal reflex depression. Because of these shortcomings, "the gallows" is not as popular as other, newer direct laryngoscopic techniques. Its apparent cumbersomeness is related directly to the experience of the laryngologist utilizing the device. Again as stated earlier, skilled hands can make it function quite adequately.

Distal light direct laryngoscopy was first developed by Chevalier Jackson in 1915 [8]. His initial laryngoscopes contained a light carrier with a tiny incandescent light bulb at the end of the carrier, powered through an attached cable-to-battery power source, and permitted direct illumination of the laryngeal area for the first time. Jackson's laryngoscopes had a removable, flat, sliding blade closing the lingual third of its circumference. This blade could be slid out, and was removed for the introduction of a bronchoscope, tube, or other instrumentation. He also completed the circumference around the distal end of the laryngeal examining tube and made this complete circle rigid and firm, thereby facilitating a view of the laryngeal anterior commissure.

Holinger elaborated on the Jackson laryngoscope design by adding a slight lift to the distal tip of the laryngoscope, permitting examination under the epiglottis for anterior commissure lesions which were possibly not otherwise visible [9]. A microscope can be used with the Holinger laryngoscope for magnified viewing; but, because of the small internal laryngoscope tube diameter, stereoscopic vision is not possible, and only a monocular image may be obtained.

This shortcoming led Jako to enlarge the circumferential diameters of the laryngoscope making it quite larger at the proximal end, and more oval in circumference, permitting that the microscope be used to its full stereoscopic capacity [10]. In addition, he incorporated two fiberoptic light bundles with the laryngoscope design to provide greater illumination for photography.

Because the tip was narrow, elevated, and close to the observer, and because of its width, thickness, and size, Jako's laryngoscope was difficult for many surgeons to use on all patients. Accordingly, in 1975, Dedo designed a laryngoscope intermediate in size between the Holinger and Jako instruments, which could accomodate the fields of vision of both eye-pieces of the operating microscope and which would thereby permit the surgeon stereoscopic visualization [11]. With this Dedo-modified instrument, if the laryngologist moves back approximately 61 cm from the patient, binocular vision is possible even without the microscope. The distal upbend, proximal downbend, and narrow midsection of Dedo's laryngoscope provide the best optical tube between the limiting pressure points, which are the upper teeth and the base of the tongue. If the surgeon moves his head appropriately, and his microscope as well, through its somewhat "hourglass" interior, it allows virtually complete visualization of the anterior commissure. Light is provided by two fiberoptic cables enclosed in a metal tube and anchored firmly in a groove of the handle. Dedo has had success in viewing the larynx directly with his laryngoscope in adults, adolescents, and even children 4–5 years old.

We have found that two light carriers, although good for photographic purposes, tend to obscure some glottic lesions as well as the subtlety of their coloration because of the washout effect of the brilliant illumination. Therefore, the Gould laryngoscope contains one fiberoptic bundle and derives some advantage from a small amount of shadow (which will often tend to make contour changes more conspicuous) and the resulting enhanced color perceptible to the examiner's eye.

Because of the variety of laryngoscopes available, the selection of a specific laryngoscopic instrument involves a certain amount of subjective evaluation. The practitioner must keep in mind that the purpose of the laryngoscope is to facilitate microsurgical care of vocal fold pathology. He must also be scrupulously careful to match the laryngoscope dimensions to those of the patient and eschew tissue trauma from an inappropriately large, or inappropriately shaped laryngoscope.

When a laryngologist is using microsurgical techniques, it is imperative that the patient's head be given adequate immobilization during direct laryngoscopy and maintained in a position conducive to adequate visualization of the vocal tract. To this end, various suspension and fixation mechanisms have been devised which assist in providing a stable operating field within a relaxed larynx.

The first suspension system was designed by Killian and was discussed in the previous section ("The Gallows"). A newer device, the Boston University Suspension System suspends the laryngoscope over the patient from an apparatus attached to the operating table. It applies force away from the patient's teeth and gums, helping to minimize the possibility of trauma. In addition, it permits examination in the Boyce-Jackson position – that with the head extended and the neck flexed on the chest – producing anterior displacement of the tongue, mandible and supraglottis – a position ideal for laryngeal visualization. The Loeb laryngoscope support is another device used to support the laryngoscope holder above the patient. Although ·it does not permit two-handed surgery, it does prevent chest movement from interfering with the positioning of the laryngoscope – a problem inherent in other laryngeal fixation and suspension devices which rest on the patient's chest.

Regardless which suspension method is selected, it is vital that the head be fixed in an appropriate position. Dr. John Kernan has demonstrated radiographically that a direct view of the larynx is easily obtained when the head is extended slightly forward. We, however, almost usually prefer the head positioned flat, and the laryngoscope fixed with the Lewy mechanism.

It is important to note that although the head must be held steady, the laryngologist or his assistant may need from time to time to exert pressure on the larynx or the thyroid cartilage to bring the anterior commissure into view.

Usually this will be a downward, gentle, steady pressure applied on the neck by the surgeon or by his assistant as the surgeon requests. No single laryngoscope thus far devised appears to be a universally satisfactory one for all surgeons or for all patients, and use of and familiarity with a variety of laryngoscopes and with their limitations is quite necessary.

To facilitate immobilization and for the patient's comfort, direct laryngoscopy should be performed with sedation and with either local, general, or neurolept anesthesia.

3. Anesthesia

a) Local Anesthesia

Concerning *anesthesia for direct laryngoscopy,* the authors use a procedure which approximates the following one: Two hours before laryngoscopy is to begin, sodium pentobarbital in an appropriate dose is administered to the patient. This drug is chosen because of its capacity to serve the dual purpose of sedating the patient, as well as that of lessening the possibility of an excitement reaction to cocaine. (Although several synthetic substitutes are available, cocaine is still a favorite agent with many since it provides vasoconstriction, shrinkage of mucous membranes and excellent topical anesthesia – all with a minimum of risk.) Meperidine hydrochloride, in an appropriate dose depending on the patient's age, size and weight, is also to be given at this time.

Application of the local anesthetic begins with the spraying of a 4% solution of cocaine or xylocaine on the lips, gingivobuccal sulcus, mouth floor, tongue and pharynx. A small pledget of cotton saturated with the topical anesthetic agent, is held in both of the pyriform sinuses for 1–2 minutes, topically to anesthetize the hypopharynx and supraglottic larynx. The subglottic and superior tracheal areas can best be anesthetized by squirting topical anesthetic agent between the vocal folds (usually 1–2 ml of 5% cocaine in aliquots as outlined earlier in the description of Dedo's technique for teflon injection) while the laryngologist looks into a laryngeal mirror. This squirting or dripping should be effected at the end of an expiration, so that the following inspiration will pull the solution further down into the airway, through the glottis and between the vocal folds. At this point it should be mentioned that the larynx is highly intolerant of foreign material on all its surfaces, and prior to commencing this application of anesthetic solutions, it is important to warn the patient that cough at least will be initiated when the solution first enters the trachea, if not a temporary laryngospasm. The aliquot dripping of local anesthetic continues (to a pre-calculated maximum dose total) until the cough reflex is obtunded, and then is stopped at that point. The earliest reflex coughs will have aprayed the anesthetic agent quite effectively on the subglottal surfaces of the vocal folds.

Recent work by DeMeester indicates that gag reflex temporarily abolished when a glossopharyngeal nerve block is effected. He uses an injection of 5 ml of 1% lidocaine into the lateral oropharyngeal wall 0.5 cm behind the midportion of the posterior tonsillar pillar [12]. This technique should very probably only be carried out in an operating room environment because local anesthetic, diffusing around the carotid sheath, may result in an occasional arrhythmia and other untoward sequences whose management may require personnel and equipment available only in an operating room environment.

To assist in suspension laryngoscopy, Calcaterra and House have devised a method of infiltration anesthesia by which profound anesthesia of the base of the tongue, valleculae and larynx can be achieved [13]. In their technique, about one hour before the endoscopy is to begin, sodium pentobarbital, meperidine hydrochloride, and hydroxyzine hydrochloride, all in appropriate dose, are administered to the patient. At the time the procedure is to be performed, each superior laryngeal nerve is anesthetized with the injection at the thyrohyoid membrane of 2 ml of 1% lidocaine hydrochloride. Bilateral blockade of the glossopharyngeal nerve is then achieved by injecting lidocaine just behind the posterior tonsillar pillar at its midpoint.

The tongue is placed in a slightly elevated position and an angled tonsil needle with 1 cm of exposed tip is used to infiltrate small increments (less than 1 ml) of lidocaine across the base of the tongue, lingual surface of the epiglottis, and the anterior aspect of each pyriform fossae. In this way, less than 10 cc of lidocaine are required to produce profound anesthesia at the base of the tongue, larynx, and pharynx.

In a very tense patient, or where a significant endolaryngeal procedure (e.g. arytenoidectomy) is contemplated, an external method for induction of local anesthesia may be used. The procedure again begins with spraying the mouth and pharynx with a topical agent. The superior laryngeal nerve is then anesthetized by making a skin wheal immediately inferior and anterior to the tip of each side of the hyoid bone. 1 cc of xylocaine or 2% procaine is then injected, at this point, into each side of the thyrohyoid membrane. In the anterior midline, just below the cricoid cartilage over the trachea, another skin wheal is made and 1–2 cc of xylocaine or 4% cocaine is dripped into the lumen of the trachea with a #20 needle.

For further sedation, supplemental intravenous medication – such as Innovar® or a mixture of Valium® and Demerol® – may be administered by an anesthesiologist. This is particularly useful during more extensive procedures (including posterior commissure work) whether an endotracheal tube is used or not.

Regardless of which anesthetic agent or which anesthetic technique is selected, it is important for the surgeon/examiner to maintain verbal contact with the patient throughout the procedure, relaxing and reinforcing the anesthetic with positive suggestions, and warning the patients if a given maneuver is expected to provoke an untoward sensation on the patient's part.

b) General Anesthesia

General anesthesia may be used to ensure that the patient is completely quiet and relaxed, and to permit adequate time for the performance of microsurgery. In this circumstance, induction of anesthesia is usually effected with intravenous agents, barbiturates, although in children, inhalation induction of anesthesia via mask is often used. Succinyl choline is then administered intravenously and continued with a 0.2% solution drip to maintain muscle relaxation, as both the surgeon and the anesthesiologist deem to be appropriate. All patients additionally are usually ventilated with a mixture of nitrous oxide, oxygen and fluorane, via the endotracheal tube, the commonest means of maintaining ventilation and additional anesthesia as well.

Several other methods of ventilating the general anesthetic patient are also available. Jet ventilation systems use jets of anesthetic mixtures blown into the trachea by transoral, transnasal, or trans-tracheal routes. In certain patients with large lesions obstructing the upper airway, however, this method does not leave enough room to place a Carden tube or even a catheter through the glottis. In such patients, an S-shaped cannula placed through the cricothyroid membrane and hooked to a conventional jet system offers a possible solution [14]. The plastic cannula may be molded into an S-shaped by hand when heated to 81.2° and when it cools, it will retain its shape. The distal segment of the "S" is placed in the center of the trachea and parallel to the longitudinal tracheal axis; the middle section lies along the neck, and the proximal section is then connected to the jetting system. The technique, although presenting a ventilation alternative, should probably not be the method of choice because it does present the hazard of surgical emphysema.

An alternative ventilating system designed by Carden *et al.* utilizes a 6.25 cm long silicone elastomer endotracheal tube with a "soft" cuff built onto it [15]. The patient is anesthetized, the tube placed approximately 1.3 cm below the glottis and the cuff is inflated to hold the tube in position. Ventilation is effected by jetting oxygen through a connecting tube. The patient passively exhales through the tube and vocal folds while the oxygen is not flowing. Obstruction to the surgical field, consisting of the 0.08 cm diameter cuff is minimal. The 25 cm diameter jet tube lies out of the way in the posterior commissure. At the conclusion of surgery, the cuff is deflated and the jetting oxygen causes the tube to be blown out from below the glottis.

Laryngeal microsurgery may also be performed without intubation according to G. E. Urban, Jr. [16]. His patients receive intravenous thiopental and breathe 100% oxygen by mask while being given 0.2% succinyl-choline intravenously until they are judged relaxed and apneic. After 2–3 minutes of positive pressure mask oxygenation has been completed, the laryngologist inserts the examining instrument. Insufflation oxygenation is established and maintained with 50–60 psi in adults and 30–40 psi in smaller adults and children. Manually controlled release of oxygen provides adequate chest expansion. In this case series, duration of insufflation in 200 patients varied from 3–40 minutes, and supplemental thiopental and succinylcholine was administered as needed.

The use of an endotracheal tube may also be avoided if a neuroleptic agent is used. It can maintain the patient in a semi-awake state and thus he can breathe on command. Neuroleptic anesthesia induction in this situation would be preceeded, of course, by the attainment of adequate and profound topical anesthesia to obtund the laryngeal reflexes.

When performing laser microsurgery, Norton *et al.* combine endotracheal intubation with Venturi jet ventilation [17]. According to their reports, a small diameter endotracheal tube wrapped in aluminium foil is used to intubate the patient after the induction of anesthesia has taken place. A gastric suction tube is then positioned to gravity-draw gases and secretions from the stomach interior, and which could compromise the immediately post-anesthetic state. The laryngoscope is inserted and the CO_2 laser is employed with operating microscope where necessary. The endotracheal tube is then withdrawn and the Venturi ventilation apparatus is placed after the anesthesiologists have inspected and suctioned the larynx clear of secretions. The jet needle is placed within the lumen of the laryngoscope, resting above the channel of the light carrier. When surgery is completed, an oropharyngeal airway is inserted and respiration by the patient is supported by bag and mask.

Other, less conventional modalities are used for the maintenance of minimum anesthesia with maximum control and these include hypnosis in its varied forms − from positive suggestion to formal hypnosis − to acupuncture which is used extensively in China.

4. Discussion

Use of *direct laryngoscopy for diagnosis* of laryngeal abnormalities is thus a fundamental tool in the laryngologist's armamentarium. Because the patient is anesthetized, direct laryngoscopy is performed in an operating room and with ancillary supporting personnel skilled in the management of anesthetic sequence and complications in attendance at all times. It is not used for casual examination, although if the vocal folds cannot adequately and satisfactorily be observed with indirect means and the symptoms require a diagnosis, direct visualization should be employed. A diagnosis is mandatory in the presence of sustained hoarseness or dysphonia in any patient and of any age. Another diagnostic utilization of direct laryngoscopy is in the performance of a biopsy, to determine the specific genesis of laryngeal pathology.

Gently aspirating surface mucus from the laryngeal mucosa with a suction tip may facilitate the location of lesions. Areas for biopsy can further be identified with the topical application of small amounts of intensifying dyes, such as toluidine blue, which will show a contrast between normal mucosal zones and areas with the broken mucosal surfaces which are characteristic of virtually all of the malignant lesions. Another facilitating device is used in a technique called transillumination, wherein an optical illuminator is placed inferior or underneath the vocal folds in order to permit that the surgeon see changes in light transmission. Transillumination can assist in determining the precise area where a biopsy should be taken.

Brushes (soft nylon or metal) can also be used during the examination to remove surface cells from the lesion and then transfer them to a glass, microscope slide so that the retrieved surface cells can be stained and evaluated by the pathologist who has a battery of staining techniques, including that of Papanicolaou at his disposal.

4*

The use of various probes and angled instruments, palpation and probing the vocal folds during direct laryngoscopy will help to identify and localize changes in surface consistency or mass or changes in the lamina propria. Small mirror and optical magnifiers can assist the examination of the undersurface of the vocal folds.

Endoscopic Surgery 4

A. Instrumentation for Endoscopic Surgery

1. Microlaryngeal Instruments

The laryngoscopes and suspension mechanisms already discussed, are added to a list of various other surgical instruments which also have been uniquely modified to suit the needs, the requirements and purposes of the microlaryngeal surgeon.

The taking of laryngeal biopsies and microsurgery itself, for example, has been facilitated by special forceps. An example of a forcep modification which has been quite helpful to a number of laryngeal microsurgeons is especially that designed by Gould. This instrument incorporates an angled control handle and uses a thumb action instead of the conventional index-finger, trigger action, which is usual with instruments of this type [18]. The distal portion of the instrument is conventional in the sense that it is a small cupped, biting forcep, a cutter-receptacle. The force required to move the cutting edge and also the force which is needed to retain specimen in the cups is transferred in the Gould instrument from the handle by a sliding rod, hinged at the distal end to the movable cutter, and also attached at the other end to the movable handle-thumb-control. The sliding rod allows easy cleaning of the instrument, and increases its durability, as opposed to the conventional sliding wire in a blind tube arrangement. To provide protection for the cutting edge of the forceps, the handle is fitted with an adjustable thumb-screw stop to limit or even stop the motion of the handle and, consequently, also of the rod which transfers motion to the cutter. This assures that the total travel of the cutting edge can be adjusted precisely to the point where the cup lips will be kept open when the forcep is not in use, and that the cutting edge will not be dulled in handling. Another feature incorporated to add to the convenience of the instrument is a forefinger guard on the stationary handle or section. This makes it possible for the surgeon to maintain a firmer grip in handling the instrument.

Grasping forceps – curved right, left and inferiorly – are also necessary for moving and stabilizing tissues while the surgeon is cutting with correspondingly angled scissors. Scalpels and knives incorporated into a small, slender blade handle also are used for cutting. These should be as small as possible and have an all-around cutting edge to facilitate dissection and deep incision. Pushing aside soft tissue, as when the surgeon is performing an arytenoidectomy, can be considerably facilitated by the use of various types of blunt elevators. Retractors are also useful and should have a special purpose guarded edge, particularly for retraction of the ventricular fold, and for adequate exposure of the ventricle itself. Suction devices of varied size must be thumb controlled, and the suction device should also be possible of employment in probing and retracting. Both open tip and closed-tip (velvet eye) suction tubes should be available and should be familiar to the surgeon.

To facilitate inspection of the vocal fold edges for small surface changes and to aid the detection of density changes, as has earlier been mentioned, a specific long, fiberoptically lit Jako transilluminator can be used. Jako has also designed other special, microsurgical tools, including a long-handled mirror which is invaluable if the surgeon is to examine the undersurface of the glottis. There are also a Jako microlaryngeal needle holder, and a surgical knot pusher.

Other instruments used in endoscopic surgical management include those devices associated with non-invasive cryogenic, laser, and electrocautery surgical techniques.

B. Cryosurgery

In 1975, Miller published the results of his work with cryosurgery on dog larynges [19]. He approached the larynx via a tracheostomy from below and into the subglottic trachea with visualization simultaneously from above by direct laryngoscopy. He found he could deliver a cryolesion capable of destroying the entire membranous vocal fold and yet preserve arytenoid motion. Furthermore, no significant injury occurred to the opposite half of the larynx or other non-target tissues – a factor related to the protection provided by approximately 3 mm of styrofoam coating these areas. S. W. Hong et al. also studied the effects of cryosurgery on canine larynges, using Brymill liquid nitrogen spray, applied either through a laryngofissure external operation, or through the Jako laryngoscope [20]. They found that with two successive 30–45 second applications, tissue temperatures below −30° C could be obtained without damage to vocal fold function and architecture – a problem common when longer freezes were attempted. They then performed cryosurgery on a 79 year patient for removal of a small ulcerated lesion on the soft palate and an exophytic lesion on the membranous portion of the left true vocal fold. The patient's voice completely recovered within two weeks, the would healed well, and after a 7-month reported follow-up period, no residual tumor was evident in the palate or vocal fold. Although, as this S. W. Hong *et al.* case history indicates, cellular tumors (including epidermoid carcinoma) are susceptible to cryosurgical destruction, it must be recognized that problems may arise as a result of the difficulty which is often encountered when one attempts to predict and determine the extent of tissue destruction that will be achieved. Due to this same tissue destruction, the use of cryosurgery precludes obtaining specimens for histologic examination during the procedure itself. In the authors' view, cryosurgery is of limited applicability in the majority of vocal tract problems which are to be treated by surgical means.

C. Laser Surgery

1. Discussion

Over the past twenty years, a great deal of interest has been expressed in the surgical field regarding the application of use of laser in surgery of the vocal tract, particularly when this modality of treatment is combined with the operating microscope. Under these circumstances, tissue which is within the viewing range of the surgeon can be vaporized with microscopic precision and accuracy. The tool has been used in a variety of surgical procedures, but its most unqualified enthusiasm is among those surgeons who use it in the application for control of laryngeal papillomatosis. When the diagnosis is unquestioned and firmly established (and taking a biopsy can be fraught with somewhat more difficulty in the case of the laser than by conventional cup forceps), biopsy specimens can be obtained. When the diagnosis of laryngeal papillomatosis is made, a marked increase of ease of management of the papillomas and a lessening of the trauma applied to the tissues within the vocal tract can result. Various surgeons have used the laser in a variety of other contexts surgically and within the vocal tract. Their use in these other parts of the vocal tract, however, does not have the unconditional and unqualified enthusiasm that use in the case of papillomatosis does.

What is a laser? The term itself is an acronym for "Light Amplification by Stimulating Emission of Radiation". The laser is a device which generates electromagnetic radiations of very specific character. Some of the other devices generating electromagnetic radiation of specific character and with which you will be familiar, are: X-ray tubes, arc lamps (as the overhead lamps on freeway systems), fluorescent lights, incandescent lights, infrared lamps, diathermy equipment, radar equipment, and radio transmitters. These are listed roughly according to their frequency ranges, with the highest frequency belonging to the X-ray and progressively lower frequencies and progressively longer wave lengths belonging to the radio transmitter. With respect to frequency, the laser with its wavelength falls roughly in the category between very long ultraviolet and long infrared light rays.

When the electromagnetic radiation is emitted or created within that particular range of frequency, this wavelength can then be focussed, reflected, refracted by lenses, mirrors and prisms, similar, in fact identical, to the ones which are used in everyday life. The particular and unique quality of laser light, however, is that in contradistinction to other electromagnetic vibrations, laser light is composed of almost completely parallel light beams, at least it is as closely parallel as the laws of physics will permit. Another unique quality of the laser light is that its emission is completely within one wave length of vibration. Nonlaser light sources emit light all through a variation of frequencies and have broad wavelengths when compared with that of the laser light source. This consequence – a very tight bundle of parallel beams of energy – is very important. Since it is a narrow range and has a very small divergence of energy beams, a small lens will thus be able to transmit all of the energy emitted by the laser to the focal point of the lens in question. This is in sharp contrast to the use of visible light, for example, which transmits to its focal point only a small fraction of the total light which is emitted from a nonlaser source.

Light which has the characteristics of being propagated in a parallel series is said to be "spacially coherent". Light which has a very small frequency spread is said to be "temporally coherent". Light which is coherent spatially and which has a narrow frequency spread is called "coherent". This coherence of both time and space leads to an intense concentration of energy and thus a reaction between matter and the electromagnetic radiation.

Lasers were first set into operation practically in 1959 or 1960, and the CO_2 laser is the one which is most commonly used in vocal tract surgery. Specifically this apparatus now consists of a long tube container into which nitrogen and helium are added to carbon dioxide, and pumped into the tube container and then evacuated, so that a certain pressure (which will be between 10 and 20 pounds per square inch) is obtained. The gases in question are supplied either from separate cylinders or mixed in the same cylinder. The reactive tube must be cooled to keep the medium in its optimum state for energy production. Then there are a series of mirrors at the top and bottom of the gas tube and an electrical discharge is created between the two. The mirrors which reflect the resultant beam of energy, electromagnetic vibrations for its surgical use are not ordinary ones. The reflective surfaces in question must be transparent to the ten micron wavelength which is characteristic of the carbon dioxide emission, and only a very few materials are transparent to this. Glass and quartz, for example, are not, but germanium, gallium, arcinite and silicon are transparent to this emission. When light of this particular wave length (10 microns) is directed into biological substances, the photons of energy can produce an intense excitation of molecular energy and heat as a consequence. The heating effects of an infrared bulb are similar well-known and probably universally experienced. This 10-micron wavelength of heat with the carbon dioxide laser is a more specific and a more intense one which is produced. This laser energy thus is capable of heating materials to an intense degree. The amount of heating which occurs will depend upon the coefficient of absorption of the tissue in question, and since body tissues are at least 80% or more water in composition, the response of tissues to the carbon dioxide laser emission are almost identical to those of water. When this electromagnetic energy impinges on biological tissue or on any substance, there is no delay whatsoever between the absorption of the electromagnetic energy and the transformation of the electromagnetic energy into heat; it is instantaneous. And because of quality of biological tissues and the 10-micron wavelength of the laser emission, the heat vaporization which can be produced is to the order of 10.6 microns radiation in human tissue per unit time of application of the laser beam. The energy in human tissue will be absorbed in 0.3 mm depths and that in turn is the depth of water which will absorb 90% of the incident energy. Because of this factor it is thus possible to separate tissues one from the other and to ablate tissue with the CO_2 laser beam, causing remarkably small damage to the tissue which one wishes to preserve. This has made possible an enormously increased delicacy and accuracy with respect to the surgical procedure [38].

Laser light is parallel, monochromatic and coherent; thus the laser light waves are synchronized and the energy of the small waves undergoes summation and creates a beam of great intensity [39].

The potential of the carbon dioxide laser as a surgical tool was recognized early and this led to the development of a laser endoscope and the stereo microscope laser attachment [40].

The cutting effect of the CO_2 laser beam on soft tissue is a result of the rapid evaporation of the aqueous cellular components. The temperature elevation of the tissue during the ablation process is sharply localized. The energy that is absorbed at the 10.6 micron wavelength acts only to increase the temperature of the tissue concerned. Absorption and transformation of the absorbed energy into heat is essentially instantaneous, while heat conduction by tissues is a slow process, relatively speaking. The temperature elevation of tissues on the average does not exceed 100° Centigrade since the cellular water is reduced to steam at atmospheric pressure [41].

The continuous wave CO_2 laser was discovered by Patel in 1964 and its surgical properties were first investigated by Yahr and Strully in 1966 [42].

2. Techniques

As to the technique of laser surgery, only a brief description will be noted here, and the interested reader may be referred to specific writings on the subject, which is beyond the scope of this effort. After the patient has been generally anesthetized, the vocal folds are visualized through a direct laryngoscope, with 10X magnification, and with the laser device in place. Manipulating the laser beam into position is accomplished with a unilateral, stereotactic control referred to as the "joy stick". The laser beam then is activated. Steam and smoke, emitted while the tissue is being vaporized, are removed with a 2 mm self-retaining suction tip clipped to the inner wall of the laryngoscope. Laser power and time settings are pre-determined based on the volume of tissue to be vaporized, and application of the laser beam is controlled with a foot switch on and off, pre-set as to depth, strength and duration of power. Laser biopsies can be effected by holding the target tissue under tension with a cupped forcep and then cleanly detaching it with several laser impacts. Although careful training is necessary to develop expertise with laser surgery, clinical results have been very encouraging, and Vaughn *et al.* have found it to be extremely cost-effective in treatment of laryngeal carcinoma [21]. When using laser beams, the laryngologist must see that inflammable materials are kept moist or protected with reflective foil. The patient's eyes should be covered, and all personnel in the vicinity should wear protective glasses [39, 61, 62, 63, 64].

D. Microcautery

Microcauterization, a technique that produces lysis if tissues by heat, is another non-invasive surgical technique. According to Kirschner, microcautery can most effectively be used for removal of exophytic lesions of the larynx as well as on patients with recurrent limited laryngeal neoplasms [22]. Instrumentation consists primarily of power application to a cautery point which is used within the larynx. Heat intensity and time duration are both controlled with appropriate operating knobs.

E. Endolaryngeal Surgery: Specific Uses

Excisional endolaryngeal surgery, whether employing indirect or direct laryngoscopic visualization, is generally used when the following disorders are present: nodes, polyps (both for Reinke's space edema and localized vocal fold polyps), cysts, chronic laryngitis, papillomatosis, webs, ventricular band pathology, vocal fold hemorrhage, granulomas and contact ulcers, carcinoma in situ, benign lesions, laryngocele or its opposite, ventricular prolapse, and vocal fold paralysis.

1. Nodes

Having diagnosed the presence of a single or a pair of laryngeal nodes, located at the vibratile midpoint of the vocal folds (or stated in another way), at the junction of the anterior and middle third of the fold, the laryngologist must then make a decision regarding the therapy of choice: whether to utilize vocal therapy alone, in combination with surgery, or to use surgery primarily. If the patient is a child, pre-pubescent, and there is no question as to the diagnosis of the organic pathology, voice therapy is the treatment of choice. Although non-surgical programs are reported and with full-time monitors of the child's voice use have yielded satisfactory results, a child in this age group often tends to misuse his voice regardless of the therapeutic method employed, Therefore, in the authors' opinion, the effort involved in such a program does not usually warrant its usage. Node surgery on children should be used only in an unusual circumstance. Examples of this circumstance would include the larynx that is very difficult to evaluate by indirect means, or patients in whom there is a question of additional pathology and in whom a biopsy and a specific pathologic diagnosis is imperative.

In the adult, a diagnosis is made by observation as well as by concensus from the results of the voice laboratory studies. The subsequent choice of surgery or voice therapy is based on several factors, including age, sex and occupation, all of which have been mentioned before. Again, let us repeat that it is particularly important to consider the patient's occupation in the light of the varying degrees of dependence the person may have on voice. If, for example, the patient is a classical, or opera singer, the risks of surgery are extreme. The tissue response to any incision, or from any surgery of even the most minute degree is scar-tissue formation – on, or in the vocal fold. This will certainly alter the mucosal wave pattern during glottal activity, probably resulting in a change in the vibratory pattern of the involved vocal fold, and possibly resulting in a change which may vary from the imperceptible to the grossly obvious and thereby change in a corresponding degree the acoustics of that particular singing voice.

Surgical Techniques

Accordingly, the authors' recommend that in the case of an adult with vocal nodules, one wait a minimum of 6–8 weeks before deciding on primary treatment. Ideally during that time speech therapy is instituted. If surgery is to be performed, the method – for instance, sharp excision with microlaryngeal cupped forcep, microcautery, or laser ablation – as well as the type of anesthesia – local or general – must be selected. Our preference is to operate on a patient under general anesthesia, using one of the direct laryngoscopes with stereoscopic magnification potential, microscope in place, the laryngoscope stabilized with a Lewy arm, placed on an appropriate supporting surface other than the moving anterior chest wall. Other institutions, however, prefer stroboscopically illuminated indirect laryngoscopy, finding therein a surgical advantage with the ongoing voice analysis which that approach permits during surgery.

Whatever method is chosen, one must take caution to avoid all unnecessary and only the most minimal mucosal excision – avoiding the resultant and subsequent vocal fold vibration pattern changes. There must be a maximal limitation of the mucosal tissue removed. Care must be taken to avoid damaging the thyro-arytenoid muscle by pulling on the vocal fold and overstretching it with grasping forcep. One must certainly avoid the tearing of mucosal strips. The subglottic area must be checked with a mirror and palpation for any further extension of pathology inferiorly. Extension here is a common occurrence and, in fact, the node itself often extends subglottically.

2. Reinke's Space Edema

Vocal fold polyps, those which are single, sessile or pedunculated lesions, are not invariably located at the vibratile mid-portion, and are often the subject of much and heated discussion. Reinke's space (or pouch) edema, however, is a variety of polyp, and is not as provocative. The etiology of Reinke's pouch edema – most often but not always in the adult and usually described as a translucent appearing edema confined to the sub-epithelial tissue layer along the vibratory margin of the vocal fold, described by Reinke, is in fact, unclear, but appears to be related both to smoking and/or to a general metabolic disorder. As the condition develops, it is characterized by an accumulation of mucoid, gelatinous fluid in the space, creating a vocal fold polypoid change which can be so extensive as to be airway obstructive.

Surgical Techniques

Surgically to treat Reinke's pouch edema, the laryngologist will usually remove a longitudinal 3–5 mm wide strip of epithelium from each fold. The vocal fold should not be stripped, however, and the removal should be a form of plication so that only the redundant edge of the edematous mucosa or polypoid change is excised. If free fluid is present, it should be aspirated. If there is fibrinoid replacement of the fluid in the space itself, excision should be limited to the estimated edge of the true vocal fold. The mucosa of the upper surgical lip thus produced should be allowed to sag over that of the lower excised lip of the vocal fold, so that approximation, although not precise, is well attainable, and the mucosal edge from above approximates mucosal edge from below.

This procedure should probably be performed only on one side at a time, since anterior webbing – webbing from the anterior to the middle-third of the opposite side – is otherwise likely. Should it be necessary to do similar surgery on the opposite side, it can be done in 3–6 weeks – a fact of which the patient should be informed prior to initiation of the surgical procedure. During this time, attempts should be made to identify the medical origin of the polypoid change. For the patient, this period must be one of abstention from smoking, an absolute necessity due to the relationship between smoking and reduplication of the pathology. A synergy appears to exist between alcohol and tobacco.

3. Vocal Fold Polyps

Vocal fold polyps are one of the most common of laryngeal benign tumors, yet developmental causes remain unclear. Their etiology appears to be associated with mechanical trauma and over-exertion of the voice, but this is not true in all cases. Additionally baffling is the frequent absence of localized inflammation even in chronologically young polyps.

Polyps can be differentiated from each other histologically, as fibrinoid, hyaline, loose or gelatinous masses. They are located most commonly along the margins of the anterior and middle thirds of the vocal fold and are variable in size, ranging from a few millimeters in diameter to sizes large enough to occlude the entire glottis. Diagnostic evaluation should include an examination of the subglottic area, where there is a great tendency for involvement. Surface tissue should also be examined for mucosal dysplasia, and to identify early malignant changes. Polyps often appears to be white or erythematous grossly, and this does appear to correlate both with age of the lesions as well as with degree of or continuity of trauma to the polyp itself over an on-going time span.

Surgical Techniques

Polyp removal is more complete, scars are less dense and less numerous, and recurrence is less common when the surgery is performed with microscopically assisted laryngoscopy than is the case with indirect visualization. The removal is most adequate when the anterior portion of the excision is limited by a small scissor cut, and the grasping forcep is used to excise the polyp along the vocal fold edge – estimating the final true edge. Evacuation is important if the polyp is fluid-filled, or of sufficient bulk, but there should be plication, to prevent the mucosal edges from falling together short of each other, or overlapping. Care should be taken, as during all endolaryngeal procedures, not to create approximating or contacting areas which will then be bare of mucosa, particularly near the anterior commissure. Subsequent web formation must be avoided, as must be the production of areas of mucosa which are tightly adherent to the subjacent vocal ligament, and which will not move freely as it must for normal vocal fold vibration to occur. Complete and clean removal of polyps will minimize occurrences, scars and voice function interference.

4. Vocal Fold Cysts

Cysts of the true vocal folds originate either congenitally or are acquired later in life. The congenital cysts are usually epidermoid, squamous epithelial lined structures, while the acquired cysts are retention or lymphatic in form. Retention cyst epithelial linings can be ciliary or glandular, or of an oncocytic nature. Oncocyte cysts, or Hürthle cell tumors of the thyroid, which are usually microscopic embryonic thyroid tissue cellular remnants, are the smallest cysts of the true vocal folds and can develop subglottically and multiply. Usually, however, they are found incidentally to other procedures, and are asymptomatic.

Surgical Techniques

Surgical techniques for excision of cysts are similar to those for removal of polyps. The laryngologist will begin by using the same principles of microscopic and stereoscopic direct visualization, and will use adequate and proper illumination. A sharp 0.5 mm cupped microlaryngeal forcep or scissors can then be used to limit the mucosal extension anteriorly as the first step in removal. The remaining cystic structure is then removed with the grasping forcep and scissors. On occasion, cysts occur deep within the vocal fold, and, in order to preserve the vocal fold mucosa, it is necessary to make a superficial, anterior-to-posterior linear incision so that the cystic structure can be dissected out gently and atraumatically and then grasped prior to its removal. Care must again be taken to reduce surgical damage, particularly when one is in the vicinity of the longitudinal thyroarytenoid muscle, the vocal ligament.

5. Ventricular Fold Cysts

Ventricular fold cysts are noted primarily in persons over 50 years of age. They are most often found in the anterior portion of the ventricular fold, probably as a result of the presence of the ductal system and the mucous gland network. They are usually mucous retention cysts and as such are frequently lined with cuboidal cells. Care must be taken, however, that there is no change toward dysplasia of the epithelium or any other early neoplastic change. Ventricular fold cysts are not common endolaryngeal lesions.

Oncocytomas, a type of benign thyroid tumor arising from thyroid tissue embryonal remnants (Hürthle cell tumor) can also be present, and may be misinterpreted as ventricular fold mucosal hyperplasia. The making of a careful and accurate diagnosis is, therefore, particularly important. In addition, to be certain that he is not dealing with a laryngocoele, the laryngologist should have appropriate X-rays made prior to surgery, for the laryngocoele is usually easily delineated by this means.

Surgical Techniques

Surgical removal of ventricular fold cysts is effected with grasping forcep and scissor as in vocal fold cysts, and entails sharp excision of the cyst from the floor of the ventricle, or from the body of the ventricular fold, itself. If the cysts lie within the body of the ventricular band, they can be removed after the surgeon splits the fold lengthwise. The exact manner of removal depends upon the size and multiplicity of the cysts. However, if both sides are pathological – as may occur with multiple cysts – both sides should not be operated on at once, and again, as in Reinke's pouch edema, the patient should be appraised of this fact early on in the management of his case.

6. Epiglottic Cysts

Epiglottic cysts found on the epiglottic lingual surface, free edge, or on the ary-epiglottic folds, can cause a sound of fullness in the hypopharynx, producing a speaking voice which sounds as if muffled, or which is sometimes described as "if there were a potato in the throat," or "a mouthful of mashed potatoes." These should again be sharply excised with grasping forcep and scissors, while the surgeon utilizes direct laryngoscopic visualization. Every attempt should be made to enucleate the cyst but occasionally and particularly, if it is unusually large, it may break. Marsupialization is then recommended with removal of most of the cystic mucosal lining, as well as the superior surface. The operation, if it is done properly, heals well and the condition is unlikely to recur under those circumstances which are admittedly the ideal ones.

7. Chronic Laryngitis

Primarily hyperplastic in nature, chronic laryngitis, including interarytenoid pachydermia, is usually characterized by generalized redness and thickening of the laryngeal mucosa. In certain cases it may deform almost the entire length of the vocal fold on the two sides. The condition can be associated with keratinization which will be seen usually as a white patchiness in submucosal areas. There will also often be nodular or localized polypoid change. As a result, smooth gliding of the healthy mucosa cover over the subjacent vocal fold body during phonation is prevented.

The etiology of chronic laryngitis has not been specifically identified, although it is known to be associated with a variety of other inflammatory conditions. These conditions include pulmonary disorders, sinusitis or other nasal disturbances, metabolic disturbances, such as hypothyroidism; or irritation from smoking, or breathing some other noxious atmosphere.

When he labels a patient who demonstrates the hoarse vocal quality which is so characteristic of chronic laryngitis, as only a chronic laryngitis and no more than that, the laryngologist is more than obligated to exclude the presence of malignant lesions. This is also true whenever an examination reveals an unexplained redness of a vocal fold. To assist in this endeavor, toluidine blue, a fluorescein stain, may be applied to indicate areas of irregularity of surface and thereby of primary concern for surgical biopsy. The only way definitively to diagnose the condition is by histologic study and, therefore, preservation of all tissue for such a study is of primary importance.

Surgical Techniques

Correction of the chronic laryngitis and voice improvement may be approached and improvement achieved surgically, provided, of course, that the suspected etiologic agent is both identified and removed. Here, one carefully removes the inflamed and thickened epithelium starting near the anterior end of the vocal fold, just short of the commissure itself, all the way posteriorly to the vocal process, in a procedure called decortication. By definition, the pathology concerns primarily the cover of the vocal fold and should not extend into or involve Reinke's space, or the lamina propria.

The edge of the vocal fold is grasped with a curved forcep (either right or left, depending upon the side involved), pulled gently toward the midline, and the surgeon makes an incision longitudinally along the vocal fold surface, to the vocal process. The mucosa of the superior surface is then cut across, near the vocal process itself. The procedure should be performed with visualization through a stereoscopic microscope. An elevator is used to raise the mucosa from the conus elasticus. If the submucosal area is violated, voice production may well be impeded and further pathology created. If this occurs, the anterior commissure will later assume a rounded configuration, as opposed to its normal angular shape, and voice alteration ensues.

As with the other procedures thus far discussed, decortication should not be performed on both sides at once or a web may occur in the anterior portion. Even though there is a so-called "safe" 1−2 mm at the anterior commissure, small strips of mucosa may peel during surgery, creating a potential for webbing. Particularly is this true in the submucosal area. Webs may occur no matter how carefully the surgery is performed and even if ablative laser techniques are used. The patient must, therefore, be warned, prior to initiating one of these procedures, that the other side should be done at a subsequent time.

8. Laryngeal Papilloma

Presumably caused by viruses as yet unidentified but possibly related to the *Herpes* groups, juvenile *papillomas of the larynx* most commonly occur in children between ages 4–6. They may be found in infants as well as teenagers. Histologically, they are identical to papillomas in adults. Juvenile papillomas are frequently found on the vocal folds and often spread irregularly across the supra and infraglottic regions, where they can coalesce to form large lesions. They can also extend into the trachea, into the bronchi and up into the nasopharynx. Adult multiple papillomata can range from a small, circumscribed mass to widespread lesions and can occur in the trachea as well. In males beyond 50 years of age, and in women past menopause, the papillomas are statistically more likely to undergo malignant degeneration.

Papillomas appear grossly to be wart-like; microscopically they are usually outgrowths of multilayered squamous epithelium, over vascular stromal pedicles. They resemble cauliflower, grape or pearl-shaped, glassy, pendulous structures. Several therapeutic modalities have been attempted for their treatment and are still being tested. These include viral vaccines derived from the papillomas, excision by laser or other means, and an experimental treatment protocol using Interferon. Surgical procedures to maintain an open airway are of primary consideration. Due to the viral nature of the papillomas, recurrences are common, particularly where mucosa is traumatised as during surgery.

Surgical Techniques

Removal consists of individually excising the papillomas along with their pedicles, with a cupped forcep or snare. The bleeding which frequently results can usually be controlled by the application of coagulants or endobronchial sponges soaked in topical adrenalin. The bleeding problem can be avoided completely through the use of CO_2 laser techniques to ablate the papillomas. According to Strong *et al.,* two laser operations, 4–6 weeks apart, are usually sufficient to remove all visible pathological signs [23]. In addition, he has found a considerable increase in the number of and time intervals of remissions when the laser was used. Whichever technique is selected by the surgeon, he must take care not to damage the submucosa and, again, to prevent web formation. The postoperative web in these patients is in some instances even more difficult to handle than the papillomas themselves, since often additional papillomas recur on the web.

Proper removal of papillomas results in adequate maintenance both of airway and voice, reduction of the tumor burden, minimization of recurrence and avoidance of the need for tracheostomy. In severe cases, however, if tracheostomy has to be performed, one should use the shortest tube possible. Patency of the tracheobronchial airway may require bronchoscopic maintenance. Tracheotomy when required for airway patency is most frequently required for infants, where regrowth of papillomas is particularly rapid. There is very little room available in an infant's larynx, unfortunately, for the performance of adequate surgery and for the removal of extensive papillomas. Due to the possibility of delayed speech development from disturbed laryngeal function, smaller children with severe cases of papillomatosis and tracheotomy should wear speaking cannulas. In some circumstances, patients with juvenile papillomatosis have shown a tendancy to remissions as well as a decrease in the frequency of reformation of new lesions as puberty appears, and the premature induction of pubescense has sometimes been mentioned in an attempt to lessen the severity of the disease process. This premature and artificial induction of pubescense is not now regarded with approval.

9. Laryngeal Webs

Webs, whether they be congenital or acquired later in life, occur in a wide variety of types. The web can be thin at the glottic edge alone or can extend extensively in the subglottic area; it can extend for only 1–2 mm or to the vocal process; it can extend from the anterior commissure to the vocal process on one side and non-symmetrically, only part way to the vocal process on the other vocal fold. Other configurations are possible. The differentiation of simple webs from glottic or subglottic stenosis, therefore, poses several problems. To exedite their separation and identification, the pathological conditions are sometimes grouped under the rubric "stenoses" or "synechiae." In any case, the primary difference is that "web" refers to the glottic edge of the lesion itself, regardless of its thickness, whereas the term "stenosis" implies both a greater involvement of subglottic tissue and that the thickening is less likely to have a mucosal surface covering.

Congenital webs are the most common congenital malformations of the larynx, and they invariably involve the vocal folds. Diagnostic, suggestive signs for the presence of a congenital web include hoarseness while the infant is crying or, if the condition is more extensive, airway obstruction. If possible, treatment should be delayed until the child is at least 8 years old and his larynx is sufficiently large to permit that the laryngologist safely perform surgery. In this way, tracheotomy may be avoided.

Surgical Techniques

Although laser ablation is used, the technique is still young: yet there is much to recommend it, both from the morbidity view, as well as from consideration of cost effectiveness. Surgical treatment is as yet relatively more predictable.

5   DHC 8 Gould et al.

Surgery usually consists of cutting along one side of the web and allowing the free edge to fold in on its base on the other side. This technique yields a fair percentage of successes and a relatively low tendency for recurrence. Endolaryngeal procedures are not always adequate, however, when recurrence becomes a problem. In this event, thyrotomy may be best, with the concomitant insertion of an endolaryngeal stent. In this circumstance, silicone film, or a metal stent (such as tantalum) to keep the raw surfaces separated until healing has occurred should be considered and the stent may then be removed. This, and other external surgical management techniques, will be further discussed in a later section.

As previously discussed, webs can be surgically acquired later in life as a sequel to the bilateral removal of lesions of the vocal folds. Scarring in the posterior commissure between the arytenoid cartilages, possibly initiated during intubation, can also lead to web formation. Laryngeal trauma, as from accidental injury to the laryngeal skeleton with fracture and shearing of the subjacent mucosal surfaces, is another consideration. Very rarely, chemical injury, or other burns of the adjacent mucosal surfaces, has been implicated. In any event, the treatment for acquired webs is the same as that for their congenitally derived counterparts.

10. Ventricular Fold Abnormalities

Ventricular fold abnormalities are less common, probably, than vocal fold pathology. Although it may be debated as to being the preferred technique, single and multiple cysts of the ventricular folds may be sharply dissected out with endolaryngeal incisions. However, a concensus seems to be emerging that laser treatment is probably most often employed in these cases, as well as in those which require removal of simple hyperplasia of the ventricular fold. Laser surgery offers the advantage of a hemostatic sealing off of blood vessels while improving healing. Simple hypertrophy of the ventricular folds may also be treated with laser if the condition is irreversible after voice therapy.

11. Vocal Fold Hemorrhage

Vocal fold hemorrhage may result from traumatic use of abuse of the voice, as, for instance, shouting at an athletic event, and also, excessive subglottal pressure applied by a singer in reaching for too high a pitch or too loud a sound. The pathology may be confined to a small area or may encompass the whole vocal fold with involvement of the mucosa due to the submucosal blood accumulation. In their premenstrual period, and because of an increased capillary permeability, females may seem to be particularly prone to vocal fold hemorrhage. For this reason, classical female singers are sometimes cautioned not to sing one or two days prior to initiation of the period, as well as the first day of the period, although there is not universal agreement on this specific issue.

Aspirin, with its known tendency to facilitate bleeding mechanisms, should be used with great caution by competitive users of voice, by singers certainly if they have previously experienced such a hemorrhage, and possibly even if they have not. Other known medications which can produce this effect include the entire group of other salicylates, as well as Ibuprofen, Phenylbutazone and some of the yellow dyes used to color foods.

Management of Vocal Fold Hemorrhage

Primary treatment of vocal fold hemorrhage consists primarily of absolute voice rest. Papain or other proteolytic enzymes aimed at helping the resolution and absorption of extravasated blood may be used. If the hemorrhage is extensive, it can be evacuated surgically, although this is not necessarily the treatment of choice [24]. Surgical excision or laser extirpation is sometimes recommended for residual small vessel enlargement, present after the hemorrhage. Particularly is this considered in the circumstance of a singer who may now note new voice impairment, presumably as the result of the increased bulk and mass of the involved vocal fold, altering subtly its vibratory quality.

12. Contact and Post-Intubation Granuloma

Post-intubation and contact granulomata are the aftermath of a mucosal (and often deeper) structural insult. Some of these insults include the use of an excessively large endotracheal anesthetic tube; the injudicious and/or heavy-handed placement of such a tube for anesthesia, or for air exchange following an incident such as drug overdose or reaction from whatever cause. Additionally, one may consider the too-long emplacement of an endotracheal tube, as in an intensive care unit, particularly if the patient's head and neck are frequently turned and the endolarynx thereby abraded by the tube. Post-anesthetic patients in a recovery room are sometimes permitted to retain their endotracheal tubes in place until the cough reflex returns and they "cough out their own tubes," obviating perhaps some tendency to aspiration of secretion and laryngospasm. This extubation technique may induce, however, still more troublesome mucosal endolaryngeal injuries even with a skillfully placed, properly sized silastic tube. Post-intubation granulomas can develop into rather large lesions. Large ones when they do occur on the vocal process, can easily interfere with airway adequacy. If there is any question that the mass is malignant, it should then be surgically removed regardless of size, the surgeon realizing that there is a tendency to recurrence. Without surgical intervention, post-intubation granulomas will usually tend to regress and often disappear within a 6 months period.

Contact granulomata occur posteriorly within the endolarynx over an injured vocal process. They are often painful lesions, particularly so when the ulcerative process involves extension of the trauma into cartilage. A high percentage of them occur in males who show a tendency to gastric acid reflux due to gastric sphincteric incompetence and/or hiatal hernia. Treatment of the

esophageal gastric hyperacidity is often definitive. Throat clearing is a frequent
contributor and must be forbidden the patient.

Psychological factors resulting in vocal abuse – apparently etiologically
associated with development of contact granulomas – are not cured by surgical
removal of the granuloma and, therefore, surgery should not be the initial
treatment. Instead, a program of vocal therapy designed to reduce patient
anxiety and alter the patient's image of what a good, efficient voice sounds like
may be instituted to achieve resolution of the problem [25]. Recently,
however, laser treatment of the ulcer base after granuloma removal has shown
some promise in promoting prompt mucosal covering of the denuded cartilage
and diminishing the cartilage pain.

13. Carcinoma in situ

In situ carcinoma should be suspected if any tissue or vocal nodule change has
been noted, or if the patient has chronic laryngitis. The area in question should
be biopsied. If results indicate the presence of carcinoma, decortication,
localized excision, or radiation therapy may be performed, depending on the
extent of the lesion and the age of the patient.

14. Benign Lesions, Miscellaneous

Benign lesions, including hemangioma, fibroma and granular cell
myoblastoma, can obstruct the airway and create vocal disorders. They can be
removed surgically, the specific technique depending on size and endolaryngeal
location.

15. Laryngocele and Eversion of Ventricle

Laryngoceles, discussed in detail in a later section, are treated endoscopically
only insofar as diagnosis, and occasionally, needle aspiration is concerned. In a
relatively unusual circumstance, virtually the reverse of laryngocele can occur,
and an eversion of the ventricle (of Morgagni) may be noted. Here, there
appears to have been an atrophy of seromucinous glandular elements, an
increase in fibrous stroma, and subsequent protrusion of the increased bulk
into the glottis, with resultant voice distortion. Endolaryngeal biopsy followed
by endolaryngeal removal is an appropriate management of the situation.

16. Vocal Fold Paralysis

Vocal fold paralysis is generally treated with teflon injection using indirect or
direct laryngoscopic visualization. An injection of glycerin may be initially
administered to preview the effects the teflon may have. This subject will be
discussed further in a subsequent chapter.

Phonosurgery: External Laryngeal Surgery Not Requiring Entry into the Vocal Tract 5

By *N. Isshiki*

In the preceding sections, it has been shown how advancement in technology and increased sophistication in the use of and instrumentation for endoscopic procedures has opened the way for the performance of operations which previously had been restricted to an external approach. At times, however, the size, location, or even the nature of the condition precludes an endoscopic correction, and in such instances the surgeon is obliged to proceed via an external route.

A. Discussion

Some of the external procedures are aimed at correcting histologically demonstrable benign conditions. Others have been devised to correct disorders in function – specific vocal disorders – and in this sense one may speak of *phonosurgery*. Many times the two categories cannot be separated completely since the anatomical abnormality can induce the functional disorder, and conversely, the impairment in normal function may lead to anatomic and histologic changes.

It should be stated that though some of the phonosurgical procedures are still in the experimental stage, others, through successful results realized in the laboratory animal, have now been performed in the human subject. We will try in this presentation to refer not only to the standard surgical maneuvers, but will focus as well on those procedures which may not yet be accepted universally. We do feel that they have the potential to open avenues for future achievement.

Let us begin by mentioning first some of the *non-invasive, external surgical procedures which do not disrupt or invade the vocal tract.* Surgical procedures in this category would include strap muscle surgery, those procedures intended to reinnervate intrinsic laryngeal musculature, surgery involving the thyroid gland, and surgery involving the cricoid and thyroid cartilages in their relation to one another.

B. General Considerations

To begin, we will first discuss *surgery on the laryngeal framework* [65, 66, 67]. The vocal folds can be conceptualized, in one sense, by thinking of them as elastic bands, suspended in turn from a mobile or deformable framework. Considered in this manner, their tension and position can be seen to be capable of alteration by reshaping the framework, thus avoiding direct manipulation of the folds themselves. This concept has clinical implications in that voice can then be considered possible of change surgically in terms of quality and pitch. More specifically, this type of surgical management is possible for diseases such as the androphonia due to the effect of anabolic or androgenic hormones, mutational dysphonia, hyperfunctional dysphonia, and paralytic dysphonia.

In the preceding chapters, it has been emphasized repeatedly that direct and wide surgical intervention on the vocal fold, per se, should be avoided whenever possible. Inevitably it leaves a scar of the mucosa, which in turn probably will' impede the vibration of the folds, and the movement of the mucosal wave. Operative intervention on the laryngeal framework is a surgical modality which is free from the problems of postsurgical vocal fold scarring. With this approach there is almost no possibility of vocal aggravation due to mucosal scarring after surgery. As a result, these laryngeal framework surgical procedures to be mentioned are practical ones and can safely be applied to a wide variety of voice disorders. They may be classified into two types: 1. Procedures which change the position of the vocal fold and, 2. Procedures which change the tension of the vocal fold.

C. Anatomy

Before we discuss any of these surgical procedures themselves, let us first consider the relevant *laryngeal surgical anatomy.* A three-dimensional understanding of laryngeal anatomy is essential for using these external surgical approaches to the laryngeal cartilages. Particularly should the relationships in distance and direction between several surgical landmarks be kept clearly in mind.

Precise knowledge of the level of the vocal fold as projected on the exterior of thyroid cartilage is of critical importance for procedures such as: 1. electromyographic examination of the vocalis muscle with an electrode inserted through the neck skin, 2. laryngofissure, 3. percutaneous cordal injection, 4. cartilage implant flanking the paralyzed vocal fold (Meurman, Opheim, Sawashima and others).

1. Anterior Commissure

In most cases the location of the anterior commissure can be projected externally on the median line of the thyroid cartilage almost at its midpoint (d–c in Fig. 19), between the thyroid notch and the lower margin of thyroid cartilage, or minimally higher than the midpoint (d–c). Individual differences can be rather great, however, for the external projection point may lie lower than the midpoint in some cases. Table 1 shows the quantitative relation between the midline projection point and the landmarks of the thyroid cartilage. But for practical purposes, it can be said that the anterior

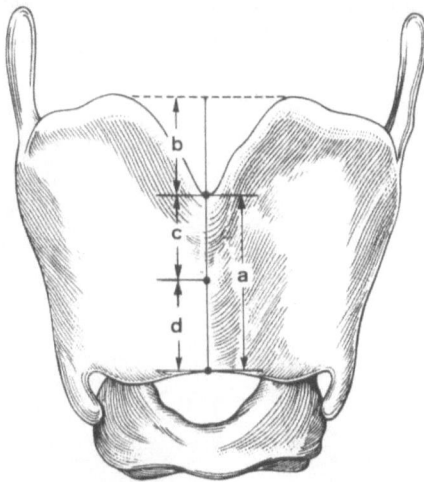

Fig. 19. Anterior view of laryngeal framework, surgical landmarks. Midway between c and d is the level of the anterior commissure

Table 1. *Projection of the anterior commissure*

Male:	Minimum in mm	Maximum in mm	Mean in mm	Variance
a	15.5	20.0	18.13	1.82
b	8.5	13.5	11.17	2.21
c	7.0	11.0	8.63	2.18
d	7.5	11.0	9.46	0.82
d–c	−2.0	3.0	0.83	1.70
d/c	0.82	1.4	1.11	0.020
Female:				
a	11.0	15.5	13.25	1.12
b	5.0	10.0	7.28	1.38
c	5.5	7.5	6.45	0.29
d	5.5	8.5	6.80	0.62
d–c	−1	1.5	0.36	0.35
d/c	0.85	1.21	1.06	0.0079

commissure may be externally projected on the thyroid cartilage at the midpoint between the thyroid notch and the lower margin of the thyroid cartilage, with a possible maximum error of 2–3 mm in the male and 1–2 mm in the female.

2. Vocal Fold

The vocal fold – its upper surface to be exact – can be externally drawn, conceptualized, or projected on the thyroid ala, parallel to the horizontal line "i" as shown in Fig. 20. Here the horizontal line connects the anterior and posterior lower margins of the thyroid cartilage, disregarding the bulge at the end of the linea obliqua. In Fig. 21 the level of the fold is shown by the 3 pins in line.

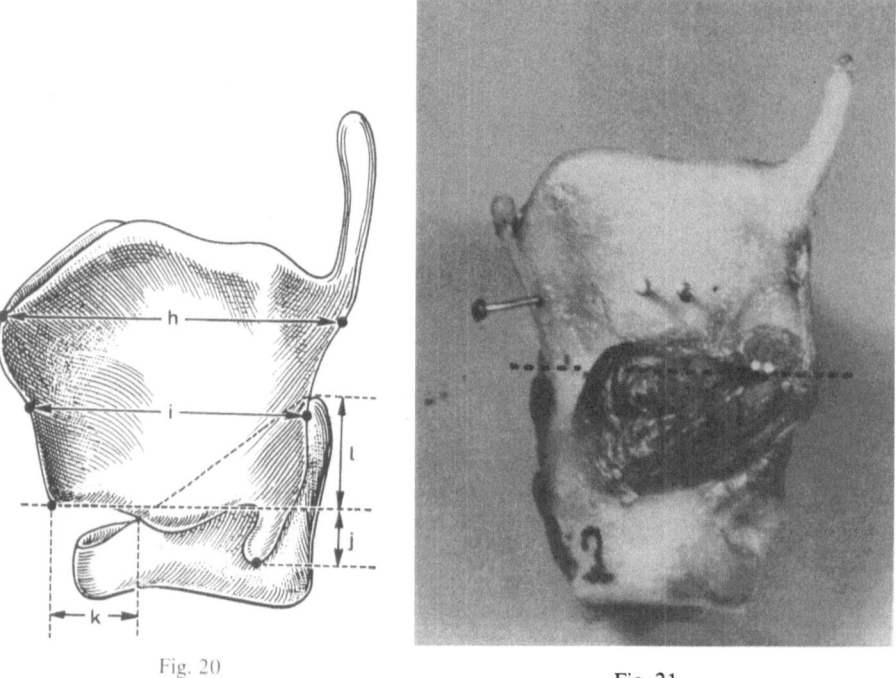

Fig. 20

Fig. 21

Fig. 20. Lateral view of larynx. The line "i" corresponds approximately to the level of the vocal fold

Fig. 21. Human (cadaver) larynx. Pins show level of glottis. Broken line indicates lower level of cricoid cartilage

3. Thyroid and Cricoid Cartilages

The thyroid cartilage covers the cricoid cartilage posteriorly. This relation should be well understood when cartilage implantation or thyroplasty type I is performed, and explains why it is difficult to displace the vocal fold medially in its posterior or cartilaginous part, by implantation procecures (Fig. 20).

4. Arytenoid and Muscular Process of Arytenoid

Knowledge of the exact position of the arytenoid cartilage is also of great importance. The muscular process of the arytenoid cartilage can be projected in the human larynx, on the extended plane of the vocal fold (Fig. 22). The

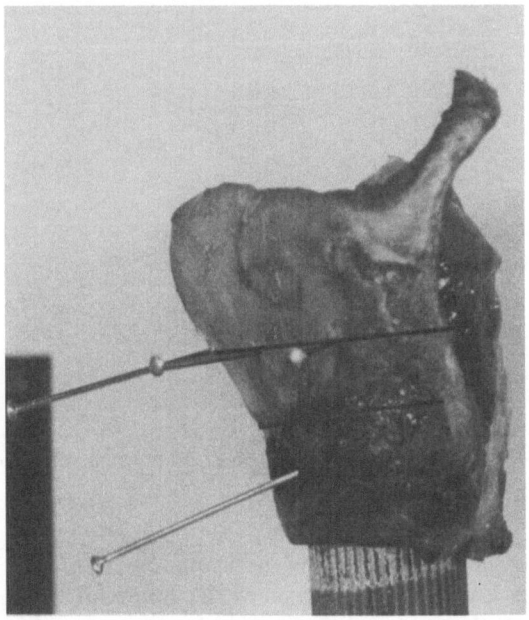

Fig. 22. Lateral view of larynx. Line drawn through the three pins, horizontally, extends through the arytenoid. Most inferior pin is in cricothyroid muscle

position of the muscular process naturally changes with arytenoid movement during respiration and phonation. The relative position of the muscular process also changes when the larynx is rotated during surgery to expose the surgical field. The posterior pin in Fig. 22, pointing to the level of the muscular process, gives a rough idea of its position during surgery.

The easiest external approach to the *muscular process* of the arytenoid is probably through the cricothyroid joint, superiorly and obliquely along the ridge of the cricoid cartilage. The distance from the upper margin of the cricothyroid joint to the lower margin of the cricoarytenoid joint averages 8.8 mm in the adult male (11.5–6.0 mm), and 7.3 mm in the adult female (11.0–5.0 mm) [68].

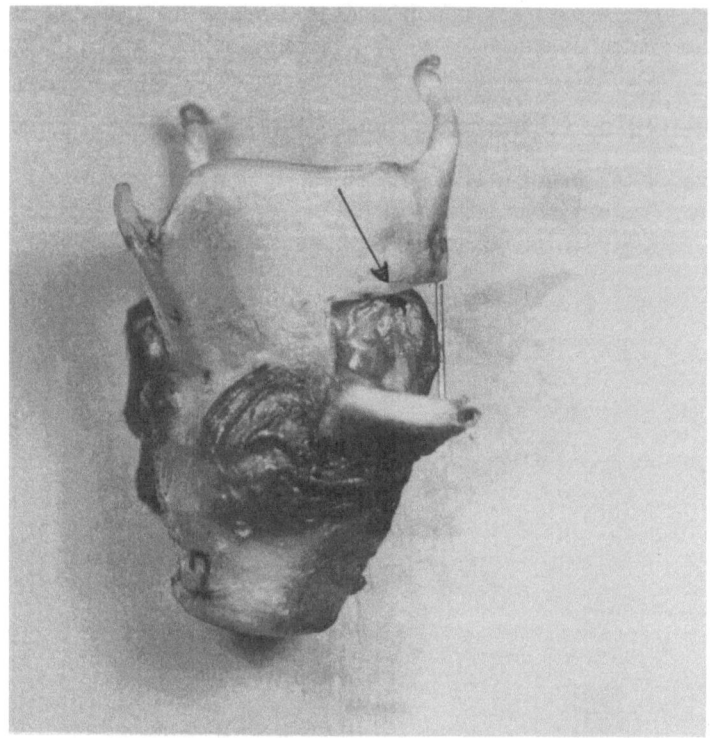

Fig. 23. View of arytenoid, with pointer toward muscular process

It should also be borne in mind that the most inferior portion of the arytenoid recess is lower still than that of the muscular process. The mucous membrane covering the arytenoid recess is, therefore, carefully to be elevated first when the surgeon is to reach the muscular process from a lateral approach. In this way, the possibility of inadvertent entry into the airway can be minimized.

Functionally, the cricoarytenoid joint is cylindrical in type. Its motion consists of a primary rocking movement around the long axis, and secondarily, a sliding one which is also along the same long axis [69, 70, 71, 72, 73].

Partly from these mechanical attributes of the joint, the vocal process moves downward on adduction and upward on abduction. The distance from the muscular process to the vocal process is 14 mm (12–17 mm) in the male, and 11.5 mm (10–15 mm) in the average female. These figures are of clinical significance when Woodman's operation (external arytenoidectomy) is performed. When such a procedure is undertaken, the sutures retracting the arytenoid cartilage outward (laterally) should be placed within those appropriate distances from the muscular process so as to avoid the suture piercing the vocal fold mucosa into the airway.

Life-size models made from a cast of the excised larynx are the most helpful tools for an understanding of the three dimensional relationships of these surgical landmarks.

Fine adjustments in vocal fold displacement are essential in phonosurgery if the surgeon is to produce the best voice obtainable. Consequently, local anesthesia is used in most cases. Neuroleptanesthesia may be used, but it must not be so profound as to suppress natural vocalization.

D. Surgery for Repositioning of Vocal Fold

1. Discussion

Vocal fold repositioning is another surgical procedure to be considered. The paralyzed fold may surgically be displaced medially in cases of dysphonia from unilateral paralysis, or laterally in cases of dyspnea from bilateral paralysis. Medial displacement is also indicated in some atrophy cases.

Medial displacement of the vocal fold, as required in patients with unilateral paralysis can be accomplished by the procedures which follow this paragraph. The size of the glottal chink during phonation is a basic factor in making a final choice of the appropriate surgical procedure. The advantages and disadvantages of each method must be weighed for the individual case.

Endolaryngeal fold injection of teflon is probably the simplest procedure and is indicated for those slight degrees of imperfect phonatory glottic closure. Disadvantages inherent in this procedure include the unpredictability of voice which may follow after injection, the relative irreversibility of result, the danger of aggravation of hoarseness if material is injected too near the vibratory margin, the possibility of migration of the injected material and the potential of foreign body reaction [74].

Percutaneous and percartilaginous injection each has an advantage in that the material tends to be injected away from the glottic margin, and the risk of vocal aggravation is much reduced. It is, however, difficult in the aged male to pierce the thyroid ala with a needle. Both are essentially procedures not done under direct vision, and require a precise knowledge of laryngeal anatomy, much prior experience and skill.

2. Cartilage Implantation for Vocal Fold Repositioning

Cartilage implants (or the implanting of other materials) offer an interesting possibility and when the glottal chink during phonation is fairly large, procedures other than fold injection may be preferred. In 1915 Payr [75] utilized a tilted, U-shaped incision on the thyroid ala to produce a pedicled cartilage flap. He then depressed this flap medially to displace the vocal fold medially as well. The amount of medial displacement is limited by pedicle length. Meurman [76] first utilized a free cartilage implant for this purpose.

Cartilage from the costal rib was inserted between the thyroid ala and inner perichondrium. Opheim [77] used an excised segment of thyroid cartilage instead, which was inserted inside the inner perichondrium. Sawashima *et al.* [78] also used grafts from the upper part of the thyroid ala inserted between the inner perichondrium and the thyroid ala through a vertical incision in the thyroid cartilage. Kamer and Som [79] utilized cartilage from the lower rim of the thyroid cartilage.

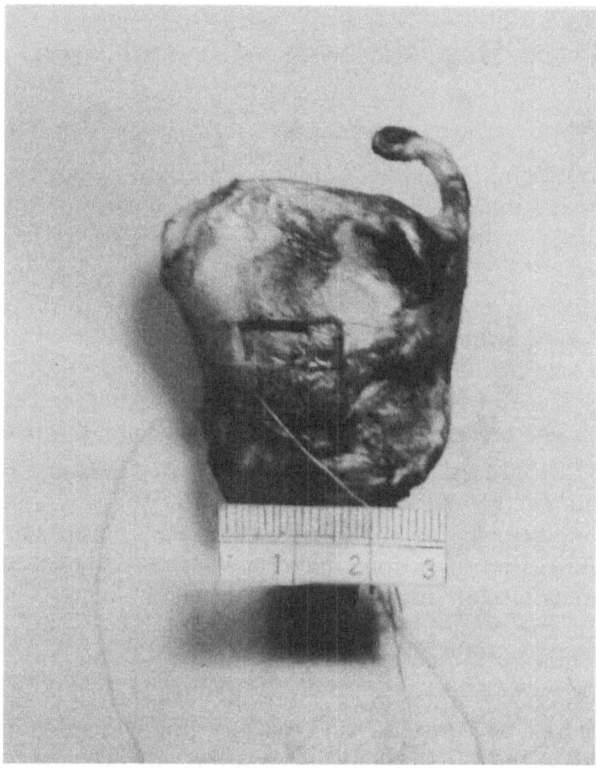

Fig. 24. Lateral view of larnyx. Framwork showing window into thyroid ala preparatory to Thyroplasty Type I

Some of the key points in cartilage implantation surgery follow, and should be kept in mind by the operating surgeon. The cartilage implant should be taken from the upper portion of the intact side. For the procedure of inserting the cartilage implant, an incision is made on the thyroid cartilage vertically, 3–5 mm away from the midline. Undermining of the inner perichondrium from the cartilage should be done carefully at the level of the vocal fold and confined just to the extent required to retain the cartilage implant. Too wide an undermining predisposes to migration of the implant after surgery.

3. Thyroplasty Type I for Vocal Fold Repositioning

Isshiki proposed a procedure referred to as *Type I* [66], which produces medial depression of a part of the thyroid cartilage. It is advantageous in that the degree of medial depression can be adjusted until the best voice is obtained. Some of the clinical tests for determining surgical indications, and for assessing surgical results may be enumerated.

When dysphonia is due to vocal fold paralysis, a meticulous history, including precipitating factors, duration of symptoms, as well as a general physical examination are mandatory to clarify if not define the specific etiology of the paralysis. These are also essential determinants in the choice of surgical procedures to be used.

Tests for Thyroplasty Type I Indication

There are several tests which are required for an assessment of the laryngeal and vocal status before and after surgery: 1. Voice recording and acoustic analysis of voice. 2. Laryngeal tomography. 3. Glottal photography during phonation. 4. Air flow measurement during phonation. 5. Manual tests (digital compression tests). Most of these have been mentioned in the preceding text.

Manual tests, compression of the thyroid alae medially by thumb and index finger, are informative in predicting the degree of vocal improvement after surgery (Fig. 25). Compression should be attempted repeatedly at various sites on the thyroid alae until maximal improvement of the voice is obtained. If the

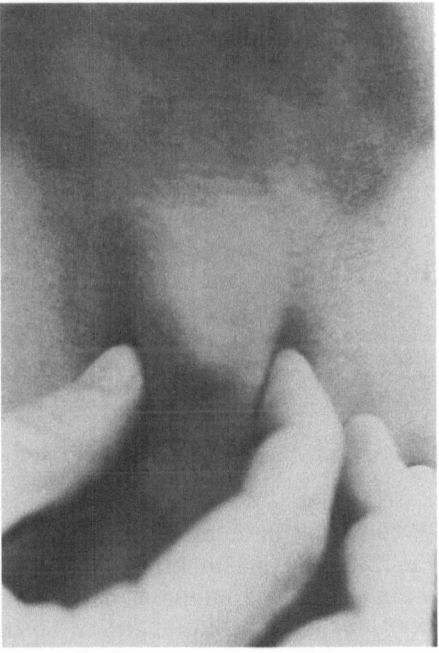

Fig. 25. Manual compression of thyroid alae

degree of vocal improvement obtained by manual compression is not as great as would be expected, there may be other problems than the glottal chink. There may be a mucosal scar or too stiff a vocal fold. The surgical results in such cases may not be as remarkable as would otherwise be expected.

Surgical Technique

The surgery for Thyroplasty Type I is performed under local anesthesia (1% xylocaine). The patient is placed supine with neck extended. An incision (4–5 cm) is made horizontally on the anterior neck at the level of the midpoint between the thyroid notch and the lower thyroid rim, as shown in Fig. 26. The thyroid cartilage is well exposed, particularly so on the involved side, by separation of the bilateral sternohyoid muscles and additional xylocaine is then injected into the thyroid perichondrium.

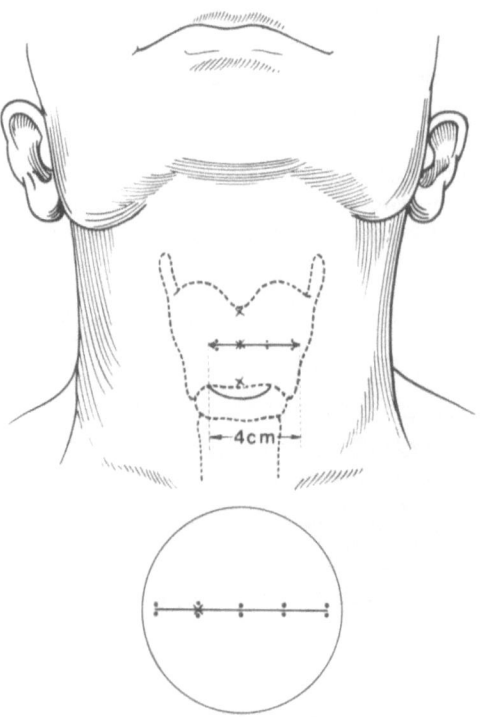

Fig. 26. Neck incision for Thyroplasty Type I

A rectangle which later will be depressed inward is drawn on the thyroid cartilage with dye. First, a point presumptively corresponding to the anterior commissure is marked at about the midpoint between the thyroid notch and the lower margin. From this point, a line is drawn horizontally to outline the upper side of the rectangle. The median vertical side of the rectangle is about 5–7 mm lateral to the median line. Generally, the size of the rectangle created is 3–5 × 3–10 mm. If it extends too far posteriorly, it cannot effectively be depressed medially (inward) because posteriorly, the cricoid cartilage is beneath the thyroid cartilage, and will block the inward shift of the rectangular piece. To incise the rectangular piece with the No. 11 Bard-Parker blade is usually easy in the female but difficult in the older male. The incision should be made very cautiously by the surgeon and with great care not to go too deeply inside the inner perichondrium of the thyroid cartilage. In this way one may prevent troublesome post-surgical vocal fold swelling.

When ossification of the cartilage is advanced, the incision is made with a vibrating saw, a rotating burr or a fine chisel. Cutting through the last thin layer is best done, however, with a knife, for this gives the surgeon more delicate control of the procedure.

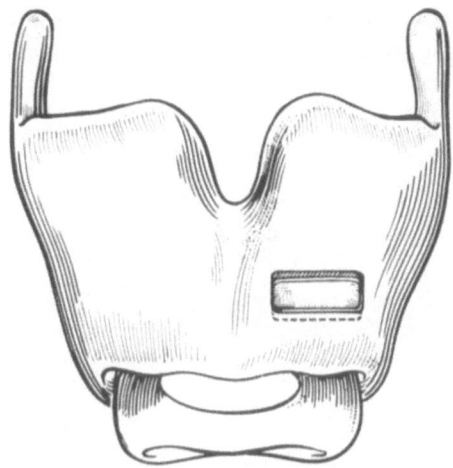

Fig. 27. The rectangle of cartilage on the thyroid ala. Usually a greater inward depression is required than is shown here

Tentative inward pressure on the rectangular piece reveals where the incision is incomplete. After the incision is completed, final separation and undermining around the margins is done gently for about a 1 mm distance. Rosen's fine elevator for the tympanic membrane or external meatus is used for this purpose. The rectangular fragment is depressed inward for varying depths to determine the degree of depression which is optimal for voice production (Fig. 27). During voice testing, one should replace the neck in the midline to avoid the distortion of voice quality which results from an unnatural neck position. Based on conclusions made from these tests, the surgeon then carves a wedge of silicone to fit what he has now determined to be an optimal depression of the rectangular fragment (Fig. 28).

Before closure of the wound is complete, the surgeon should undertake manual cricothyroid approximation to find if this maneuver can still further improve the voice. It is known from dog experiments that cricothyroid approximation displaces the vocal cord caudally by 1 mm on the approximated side; therefore, testing should always be tried and done when the paralyzed fold is positioned higher than its innervated opposite. If the manual compression procedure does improve voice, two 3–0 nylon sutures are used to draw the cricoid cartilage toward the thyroid cartilage. In passing the suture through the thyroid cartilage near the median line, the surgeon should take care not to pierce the inner mucosal lining. The soft tissue between the cartilage and the mucosa will be found to be very thin near the anterior commissure. On the exterior of the thyroid cartilage, bolsters made of cartilage or silicone are to be used between the cartilage surface and the surgical knots. For cosmetic reasons, the wound should be closed carefully with 4–0 nylon buried sutures and 6–0 adaptation sutures. To minimize the development of a hypertrophic scar, local compression with sponges and restriction of neck motion for a while with a collar corset may be recommended.

Slight edema of the involved vocal fold may last for a week or so but never to the extent of causing stridor or dyspnea. Voice rest is recommended at least for a week.

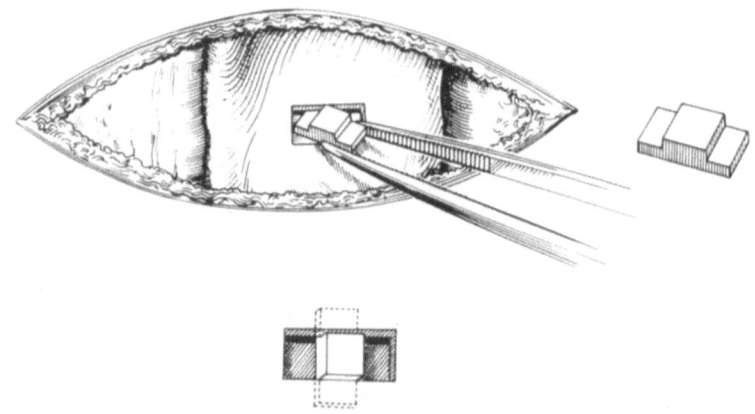

Fig. 28. Silicone is shaped and then wedged beneath the ala

4. Arytenoid Adduction or Rotation for Vocal Fold Repositioning

Discussion and Anatomy

Let us now consider another procedure, that of arytenoid adduction or rotation [80]. When the glottal chink is large and the paralyzed fold is indeed situated higher than the intact and normally innervated one [81], the surgical procedures mentioned earlier are usually insufficient to reduce both the glottal chink and the level differences between the two folds. Arytenoid adduction is indicated in these cases.

Aryntenoid adduction similar to that induced by contraction of the adductor muscles during normal phonation can be approximated surgically by pulling the muscular process anteriorly with nylon sutures, and in line with the adductor muscles. This simulated arytenoid adduction effectively reduces the glottal chink as well as reducing the difference in level between the two folds.

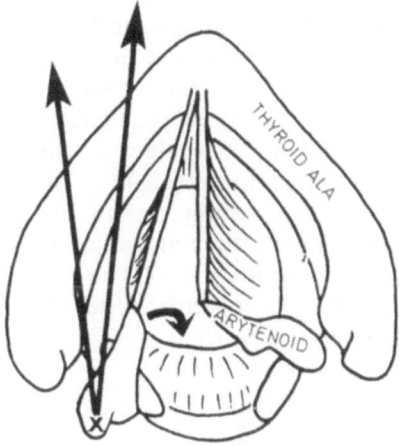

Fig. 29. Traction vectors for pull on arytenoid cartilage, rotating the vocal fold medial and caudal

Surgical Technique

To summarize, arytenoid adduction is accomplished surgically by placing traction on the muscular process with two 3−0 nylon sutures tied in the approximate direction of the lateral cricoarytenoid and lateral thyroarytenoid muscles (Fig. 29). Vocal improvement after this type of surgery is often quite dramatic.

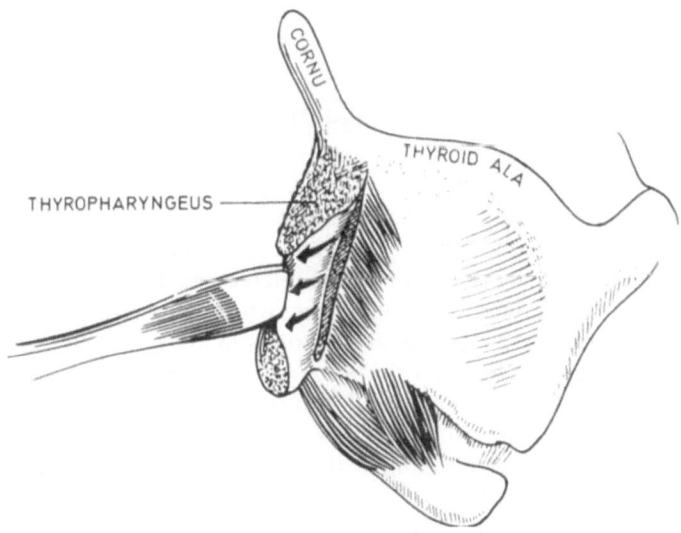

Fig. 30. The posterior margin of the thyroid cartilage is exposed

This surgery is performed under local anesthesia. The patient is placed supine, with the head extended and rotated toward the intact side. A skin incision is made horizontally on the paralyzed side at the level of the midpoint between the thyroid notch and lower margin of the thyroid cartilage as shown in Fig. 15. If the patient has an incisional scar from previous surgery in the area, the entry incision may be made there, cosmetically excising the scar at the same time. The thyroid cartilage is exposed laterally down to the posterior margin. The thyropharyngeal muscle is elevated and sectioned to free the posterior margin of the thyroid cartilage (Fig. 30). Subperichondrial elevation is continued around the thyroid margin and to the interior surface of the thyroid ala. The cricothyroid joint is then dislocated to produce a wide surgical field (Fig. 31). The mucous membrane of the pyriform recess is turned superiorly in continuity with the superichondral elevation. Care should be taken not to enter the airway.

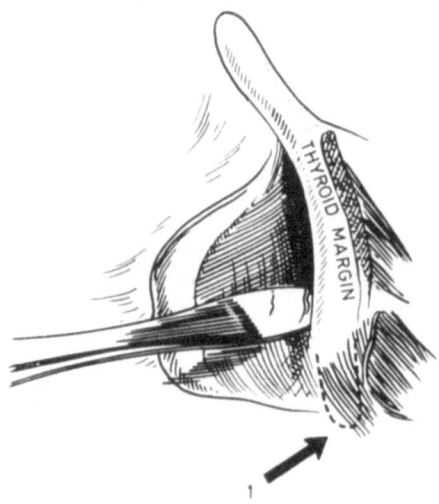

Fig. 31. The cricothyroid joint is dislocated. The arrow points out the cricothyroid joint

Approach to the muscular process starts with identification of the surface of the cricothyroid joint (B in Figs. 32 and 33). If one proceeds from this point obliquely upward along the ridge of the cricoid cartilage, the muscular process is visualized. It produces a prominence whose presence is confirmed with digital palpation (Fig. 34). A small incision is made at the end of the posterior cricoarytenoid muscle to open the joint. The brilliant white joint surface can now be seen as a final anatomical confirmation (Fig. 35). Two 3–0 nylon sutures are tied across the muscular process. They should incorporate a sufficient amount of soft tissue near the muscular process to cushion the force of traction (Fig. 36).

These same sutures are then passed through the thyroid ala, one laterally and the other more medially, with the use of a large, gently curved needle. In

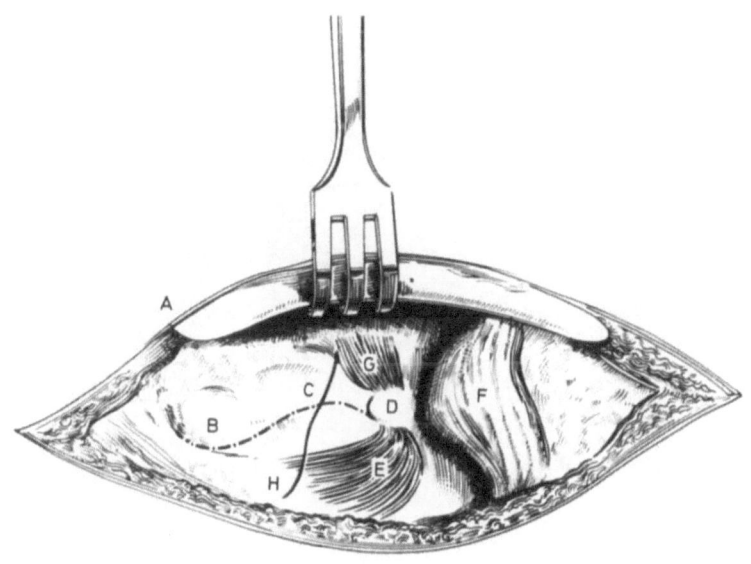

Fig. 32. Operative field for arytenoid cartilage. *A* Thyroid cartilage. *B* Surface of cricothyroid joint on cricoid cartilage. *C* Ridge between lateral and posterior surface of cricoid. *D* Muscular process. *E* Posterior cricoarytenoid. *F* Mucosa of pyriform recess. *G* Lateral cricoarytenoid. *H* Branch of recurrent laryngeal innervating adductors

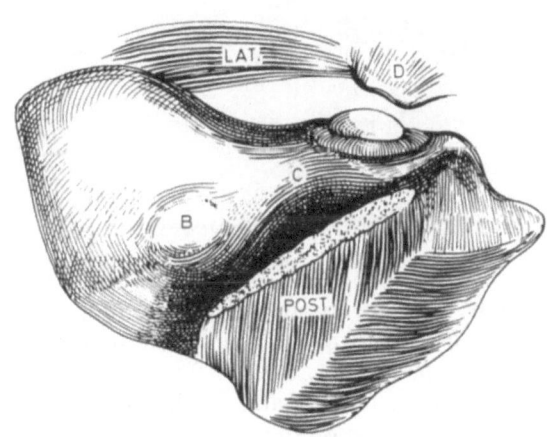

Fig. 33. View of arytenoid prominence. *LAT* Lateral cricoarytenoid muscle. *POST* Posterior cricoarytenoid. Cricoarytenoid joint *(D)* can be reached from *(B)* via *(C)*

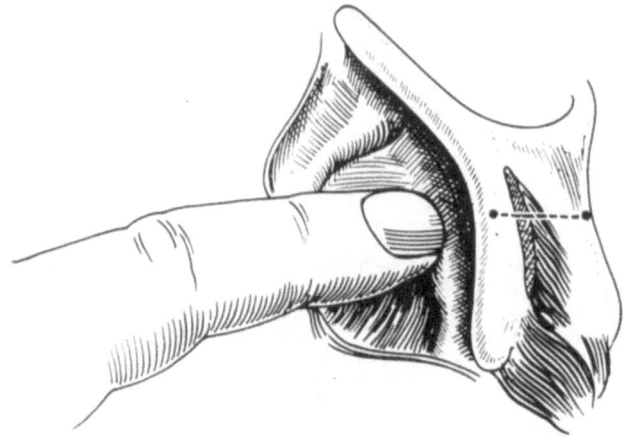

Fig. 34. Digital palpation of arytenoid

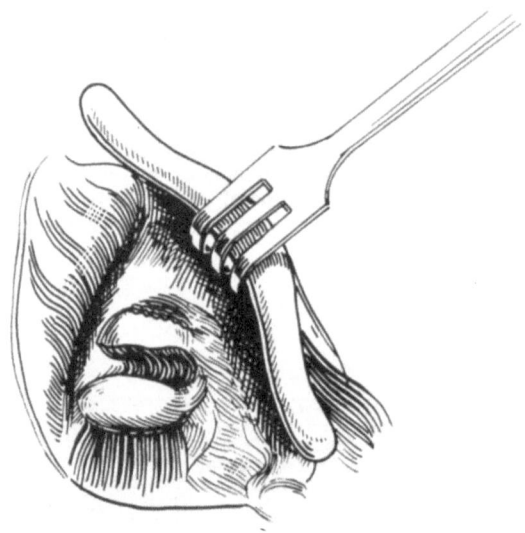

Fig. 35. Exposure of cricoarytenoid joint

the aged male patient with advanced ossification of the thyroid cartilage, drilling through the cartilage to produce a tiny hole may be necessary so that the suture needle can be passed.

The patient is then asked to phonate, as the surgical team assesses the effect of the first tentative traction on the sutures. Too much adduction usually results in a strenuous, squeezed, rough voice. Too breathy a voice may be produced if the traction sutures are positioned too anteriorly, for a traction force which is made parallel to the length of vocal fold will produce shortening and relaxation.

It is important that the sutures not be tied with excessive tension. A bolster is not required on the thyroid ala because final suture tension should not be great. A drain is inserted inside the thyroid ala and retained for two to three days to reduce postoperative swelling of the arytenoid recess. Postoperatively, swelling in the arytenoid recess usually lasts for a one or two week period and should require no specific treatment. Vocal rest is recommended for at least a week. Marked improvement in voice can be expected when arytenoid adduction is used in cases experiencing a severe dysphonia due to unilateral paralysis. If the paralyzed vocal fold is accompanied by scarring, as often results from laryngeal trauma, the prognosis for good voice is rather poor.

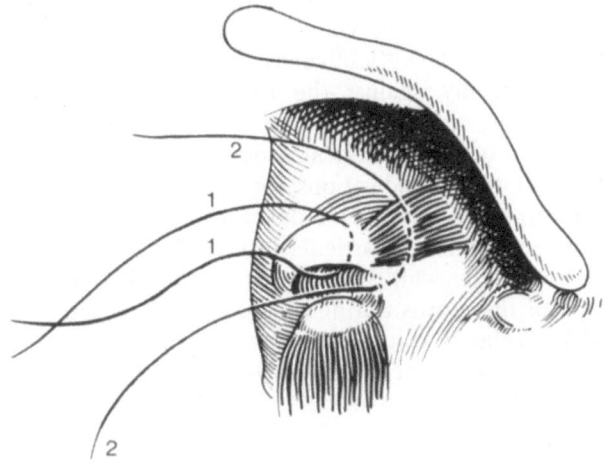

Fig. 36. Sutures 1 and 2 to reposition arytenoid.
2 grasps primarily the lateral cricoarytenoideus

E. Surgery for Vocal Fold Tension Change

1. Theoretical Basis

We may now proceed to a consideration of those *surgical procedures which change tension of the vocal fold* [65, 67, 68, 83]. Theoretically, three factors are involved in changing vocal pitch: mass (thickness of the vocal fold), stiffness (tension), and length. These may be likened, somewhat to the mechanisms for pitch control in the violin: pitch can be raised by shortening the vibrating string, making the string more tense, or by using a thinner string.

Vocal fold tension also increases as pitch rises. This increase in tension is accomplished mainly by contraction of the cricothyroid muscle. In extremely high pitch ranges (falsetto), mass control (decrease in mass) becomes effective.

High-pitched mutational voice may be explainable by a very tense fold, which either can be on a functional or on an organic basis. The voice which follows irradiation, or laryngeal trauma is often very high in pitch, probably because of the resultant scarring, which makes it very stiff. The voice in laryngeal web, where there will be a short effective length of the vocal fold, is generally high-pitched as well as hoarse.

2. Discussion

There are *surgical procedures designed to raise vocal pitch,* and we may discuss them at this time. We must, however, recall that all these procedures relate not only to pitch, but also to vocal quality as well. Some of the procedures may result in an increased difficulty in voice production and predispose to the development of an aphonia. The effectiveness of surgery in raising vocal pitch should be weighed carefully against the risks of producing dysphonia or aphonia.

If we first take note of those surgical procedures to raise vocal pitch, we must first give thought to the indications for surgery of this sort. The most frequent is the androphonia which can develop after the administration of anabolic or androgenic hormone, particularly to the young female. The vocal folds appear thick and rather whitish without signs of inflammation, and there is imperfect closure of the glottis during phonation. This type of surgery may also be indicated for related voice disorders due to hormonal diseases, for paralysis of the cricothyroid muscle, for the transsexual, or as a rejuvenation procedure for the aged woman.

3. Surgical Approximation of Cricoid and Thyroid Cartilages

Approximation of the cricoid and thyroid cartilages by suture [65, 67, 68, 82, 83] (Fig. 37) is the only method which can raise vocal pitch without risk of deterioration in voice quality. It is a type of surgery on the laryngeal framework, and generally is much safer than direct intervention on the vocal fold, in terms of possible postoperative aggravation of voice quality. This type of surgery does have a drawback though, in that there is a limitation to the extent to which vocal pitch can be elevated. Again, to ·use the admittedly imperfect violin analogy, the highest tone which can be produced with a thick string is limited, no matter how much tension is placed on that string. Another liability is that this type of surgery will also reduce the range of pitch variation. Various tests to measure pitch level for sustained vowel production and speech, and the vocal pitch range, are required before surgery of this sort, and manual compression testing is essential to verify the indication for surgery.

Manual Testing

The cricoid and thyroid cartilages are approximated bimanually during sustained phonation to see how much this maneuver can elevate vocal pitch (Fig. 38). If the pitch increment is substantial and if the patient is satisfied with

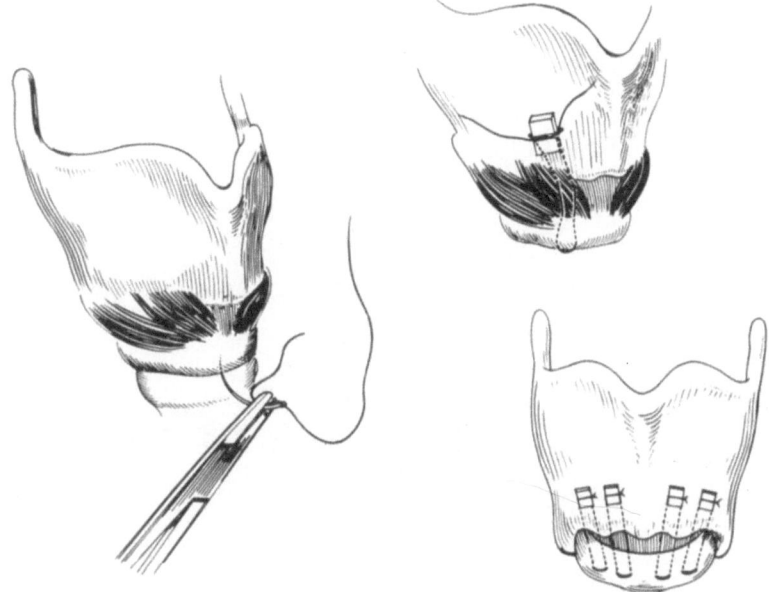

Fig. 37. Approximation of thyroid and cricoid cartilages

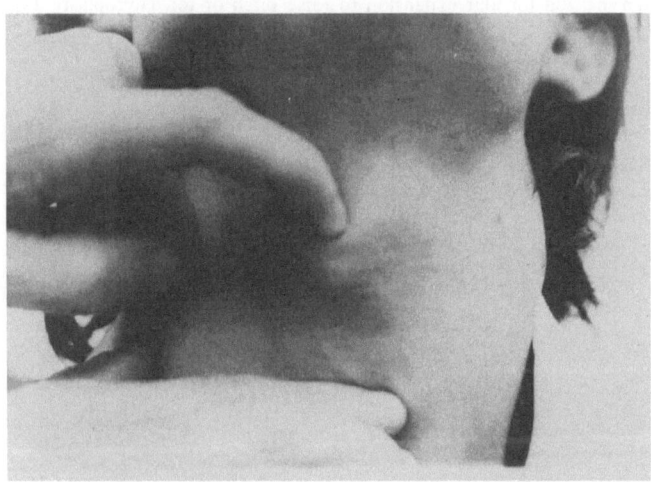

Fig. 38. Manual approximation of thyroid and cricoid

the extent of pitch increase produced by manual manipulation, surgery in the form of cricothyroid approximation may be indicated.

Technique for Cricothyroid Approximation Surgery

Surgery is done under local anesthesia. The patient is again supine with neck extended. An incision is made horizontally at the level of the lower rim of the

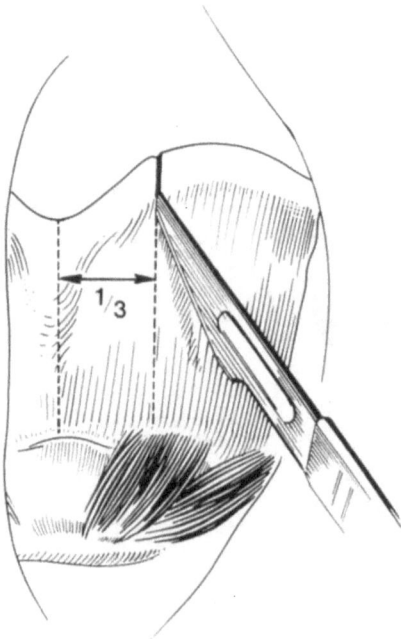

Fig. 39. Cartilage incision for alar expansion to raise pitch or for Thyroplasty Type III to lower pitch

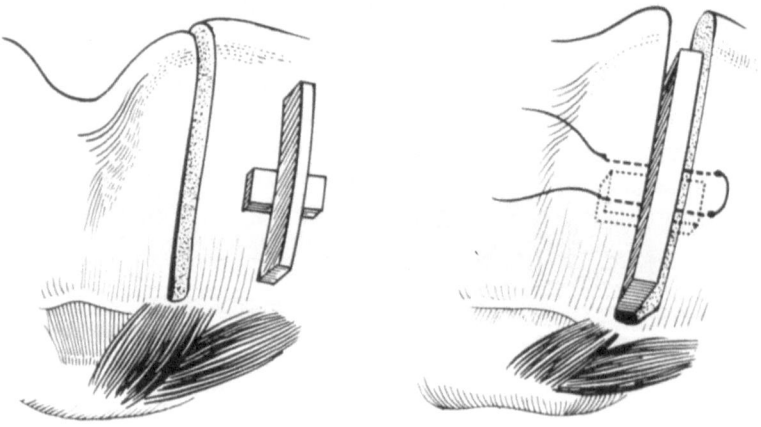

Fig. 40. The thyroid alar split is wedged apart, horizontally

thyroid cartilage. The thyroid and cricoid cartilages are exposed and 3−0 nylon interconnecting sutures, two for each side, are passed through the cartilages (Fig. 37). The suture is first passed through the cricoid cartilage from below upward and withdrawn at the site where the cricothyroid muscle attaches to the cricoid cartilage. It is then again passed beneath and through the thyroid cartilage. A bolster, made of silicone or a cartilage fragment, is necessary on the thyroid cartilage to cushion against the tension produced (Fig. 37). Care should also be taken not to pierce the mucosal lining, when passing the suture through the median part of the thyroid cartilage.

After all four sutures are passed and are ready to be tied, the pillow beneath the neck is removed. This positional change will permit a test of thyroid approximation upon vocal pitch with the head and neck conventionally aligned, in a comfortable posture. The patient is asked to phonate while the cricoid and thyroid cartilages are approximated. When the suture is finally tied, an assistant lifts the cricoid cartilage toward the thyroid cartilage. The two paired sutures are then tied alternately, left and right maintaining an equal approximation for both sides. Cricothyroid distances before and after surgery are measured and recorded for subsequent reference.

4. Lengthening of Vocal Fold

Discussion and Technique

Antero-posterior lengthening of the thyroid ala [68] (Figs. 39, 40, 41] results in an anterior shift of the anterior commissure, and a consequent lengthening

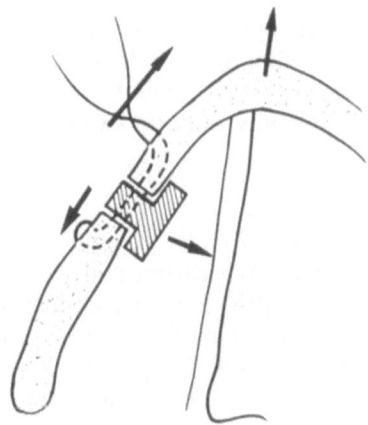

Fig. 41. Antero-posterior lengthening of the thyroid ala. The effect is an elongation and slight medial displacement of the vocal fold

(tensing) of the vocal fold. Cartilage fragments, or shaped silicone may be interposed in the vertical slit produced on the thyroid ala. So far as the present authors' experience is concerned, the efficacy of this type of surgery in elevating pitch is not as great as that obtained by cricothyroid approximation. An outline of the surgical procedure has already been illustrated. A vertical incision in the thyroid ala is made (Fig. 39), producing a slit into which a silicone plate is to be inserted, expanding the ala antero-posteriorly.

5. Increase in Stiffness of Vocal Fold

Discussion

Scarification [83, 84] is or may be intentionally produced on and/or in the vocal fold to increase stiffness of the fold. Superficial longitudinal shavings off of the mucosa, or deep longitudinal incisions (parallel to the vibratory margin) are the two possibilities. The resultant effectiveness of this procedure in elevating pitch will greatly depend upon the site and extent of scar produced. If scar is produced near the vibratory margin, the effect in elevating pitch would appear to be great, although the risk of deterioration in voice quality would likewise be great. Generally speaking, scar on or in the vocal fold impedes mobility of the mucosa, a very important factor in vocal fold vibration. Furthermore, if the folds are stiff, a higher subglottal pressure will be required to drive them into vibration. Considered from this view-point, the choice of a surgical procedure designed to produce scar should be made rather hesitantly as a primary measure, in an effort to avoid deterioration of voice quality or difficulty in voice production. After at least a six-month follow-up period, a second operation to augment the scar may be considered if the effect is not satisfactory.

Indication

This type of surgery is indicated for the excessively low-pitched voice in females as mentioned in the preceding section. If the voice is extremely low or if the patient wants to raise pitch to a great extent, longitudinal scar production may be indicated rather than cricothyroid approximation.

Technique

Surgery for this purpose is performed under general intubation anesthesia or neuroleptanalgesia. A laryngoscope is inserted and the patient suspended to obtain a good, stable view of the glottis. One or two deep incisions usually are made in each of the vocal folds. A special fine knife is used with microscopic surveillance. Incisions are placed parallel to, and 1–3 mm apart from the vibratory margin. The surgical result can be evaluated only after a period of one year or so postoperatively.

6. Other Techniques for Increasing Tension of Vocal Fold

Other types of surgery to raise pitch include reduction cordoplasty and anterior adhesion technique (web formation) but these are to be examined further by experimental procedures before they may be applied to human subjects. In these procedures, the possibility of developing a severe breathy dysphonia after surgery is theoretically rather great, and the necessity for raising pitch should be well-weighed against these possible undesirable side-effects before the choice for surgery is made.

7. Decreasing Tension of Vocal Fold

a) Theoretical Basis and Discussion

Pitch-lowering surgical procedures are described more commonly [65, 67, 68, 82, 83]. Most frequently as choices for surgery of this variety are the so-called mutational voice dysphonias. Other indications include the excessively high-pitched voice in the male which may occur as a result or symptom of laryngeal trauma, irradiation, laryngeal web, or vocal fold atrophy which may also occur in some type of hyperfunctional dysphonia. Before surgery is elected as a treatment of choice, it should always be kept in mind that excessively high pitch can be temporary, reversible, functional, or psychogenic and may well be responsive to voice therapy and/or psychological treatment. Conservative treatment should be tried for at least three months to ascertain the value of a non-surgical approach.

It must also be stated, however, that in many instances, the psychological aspect has been over-emphasized in cases of high-pitched voice in the male. These patients are often diagnosed as having a mutational voice disorder without definite, positive evidence that a disturbance of one of the normal developmental processes actually has caused the high-pitched voice to be a continual one from childhood to the present. The diagnosis itself implies that psychological factors must be responsible for the excessively high-pitched voice; but it is obvious that not all of these so-called mutational voice disorders are psychogenic, and thereby approachable with vocal or psychological treatment. In this sense, "mutational voice disorder" may be a kind of wastebasket term, which includes a variety of clinical entities. These patients should be further classified on the basis of laryngeal findings, the results of various tests, and the effect or lack of effect of treatment.

Surgical possibilities for patients with these disorders are more predictable. Again, in analogy to the violin string, the voice can theoretically be lowered in pitch by 1. relaxation of the vocal fold, 2. increase in mass (augmentation cordoplasty), and 3. elongation of the vocal fold.

Surgical elongation of the vocal fold without changing tension is impossible except in the case of laryngeal web. Here, web incision produces an increase in effective length without a change in tension.

Augmentation of the vocal fold, which theoretically should lower pitch is also troublesome, for it will greatly hinder mobility of the covering mucosa, and consequently impede the glottic vibratory patterns. Too much surgical intervention on, or in, the vocal fold will create scar. This scar in turn will work as a factor to raise pitch, counteracting the aims of surgery. If too much mass is injected into the fold in order to lower pitch, the injected portion may not vibrate at all. As a consequence, only the small, narrow portion along the vibratory margin on the median side of the injected site may vibrate. This can, in effect, decrease the vibrating mass, again raising the pitch in contradiction of the aims of the original surgical intent.

Logically, and in most cases, surgery on the laryngeal framework is the procedure of choice to relax the vocal fold. The manual compression test, digitally pressing inward on the cricothyroid membrane while the patient phonates, is helpful to delineate an indication for surgery. Injection of a local anesthetic into the cricothyroid muscle may also be tried to find whether or not a temporary paralysis of that muscle lowers pitch. If it does, the high pitch is more likely to be hyperfunctional in origin and speech therapy should be initiated as a first choice of procedure.

b) Thyroplasty Type III: Technique

Thyroplasty Type III [65, 82, 83], or shortening the antero-posterior distance of the thyroid ala by means of a vertical strip excision of cartilage is predictable surgically. In this procedure, and with local anesthesia, an incision is made horizontally on the neck to expose the thyroid ala. Two vertical, parallel incisions, 1–2 mm apart from each other, are made on the ala to remove a vertically oriented, long rectangular piece of cartilage. After the cartilage strip is excised one may test its effect on pitch. Subluxation of the lateral side of the incised ala beneath the median side may prove to be more effective in lowering pitch and in obtaining better voice quality in some cases. Variations in the relationships of the incised margins of the ala should be tried to obtain the best voice (Fig. 42/1–4).

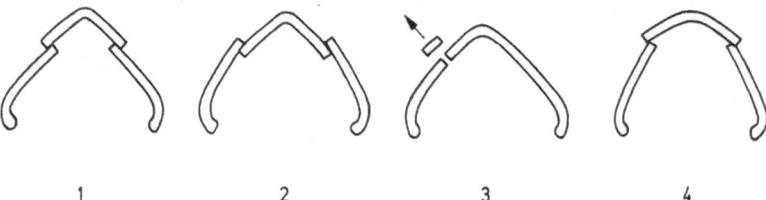

1   2   3   4

Fig. 42. Variations capable of trial in Thyroplasty Type III for lowering pitch, or for relaxing a spastic glottis

Once a satisfactory result is obtained, the sectioned alar margins are fixed in that position. If the effect of lowering pitch is insufficient despite the various combinations of alar reconstructions which are tried and tested, shortening on the contralateral ala is added (Fig. 42/3). Usually, however, shortening of the unilateral ala is sufficient, and no irregular vibration of the fold occurs, even though the two are asymmetrical in tension, as demonstrated both experimentally and clinically [85].

c) Sectioning of Superior Laryngeal Nerve or Cricothyroid Muscle

In any consideration of external laryngeal surgery, section of the superior laryngeal nerve may be indicated in a very limited series of cases, including excessively high pitch, or some types of spastic dysphonia. The effectiveness of sectioning the unilateral superior laryngeal nerve can roughly be evaluated by the injection of a local anesthetic (1% xylocaine) about the nerve or into the cricothyroid muscle. If the anesthetic injection improves the voice to the patient's satisfaction, an indication for this technique may exist. This particular technique has been utilized in patients with mutational voice disorders, with satisfactory results [68]. After Thyroplasty Type III, or the vertical strip excision technique had been developed for lowering vocal pitch, however, section of the superior laryngeal nerve and/or the cricothyroid muscle was no longer considered as strongly.

Technique

A surgical technique for superior laryngeal nerve section is as follows: The thyroid and cricoid cartilages are exposed using local anesthesia. Anesthetic is injected into the unilateral cricothyroid muscle under direct vision. After one secures confirmation of vocal improvement, the cricothyroid muscle fibers are cut sufficiently to suppress their function. Bilateral section of the superior laryngeal nerve is contraindicated in any case. After unilateral cutting of the cricothyroid muscle, injection of anesthetic into the contralateral cricothyroid muscle will result in a very rough, hoarse voice resembling that of glottal fry. It is assumed that the rough, extremely low-pitched voice is produced by too flaccid a vocal fold.

Vocal improvement obtained by unilateral section of the cricothyroid muscle may be ascribed to relaxation of the too tense vocal fold. Improvement may also partly by ascribed to slight abduction of the vocal fold which adducted too much for proper glottal closure. Somehow, blocking the proprioceptive feedback mechanism by section of the nerve or muscle may also be involved. The disadvantages of nerve or muscle section are: 1. control of pitch decrement is difficult, 2. pitch variation will be reduced by unilateral N-M section. In the *Thyroplasty Type III,* the function of the cricothyroid muscles to vary the vocal pitch is retained.

d) Sectioning of Recurrent Laryngeal Nerve

According to Dedo, sectioning the recurrent laryngeal nerve may provide dramatic relief to a patient suffering from spasmodic dysphonia [26]. The condition itself has previously been attributed exclusively to psychogenic factors [27]. More recent work, including that of Dedo and of H. Tucker, may indicate that its etiology may be associated with disturbances in the proprioceptive (neurological) control of the vocal folds. Clinical symptoms of spastic dysphonic vary but include weak, tight-sounding phonation which results from the vocal folds being excessively adducted. Together with these possibly incoordinate contractions, face and neck grimaces and eye blinking often accompany the affliction, as in Meige Syndrome.

Observation of the fact that the vocal fold retracts to a paramedian position in subjects suffering from recurrent nerve paralysis suggested to Dedo that a deliberate induction of nerve paralysis, by nerve sectioning, might provide relief to patients with spastic dysphonia. He tested this hypothesis by inducing temporary paralysis with an injection of 1% lidocaine, adjacent to the cricothyroid joint, and in appropriately selected patients he noted a significant improvement in voice when paresis of the recurrent nerve ensued. Surgery is usually performed only when significant vocal improvement is noted after injection, and vocal fold paresis is seen.

Surgical Technique   ·

The surgery is performed under local or general anesthesia depending on the preference of the surgeon via a collar incision, one fingerbreadth below the cricoid cartilage. The dissection is extended down the anterior tracheal surface and around its right side to the tracheoesophageal groove. Once identification of the recurrent nerve (1 cm lateral to the trachea at the level of the inferior pole of the right thyroid gland) is secure, an assistant stimulates the nerve while the glottis is observed through a direct laryngoscope. The structure is presumed to be the entire recurrent nerve if the vocal fold contracts abruptly at the instant of stimulus. If this is the case, it is ligated with a silk ligature and a 1 cm segment is removed adjacent to the inferior pole of the thyroid gland approximately 3–4 cm below the cricoid. Gut subcutaneous sutures and Steri-strips are used to close the incision, and a drain is kept in place.

To date, of 200 spastic dysphonic patients who underwent recurrent laryngeal nerve section, 72 have been evaluated 1–3 years postoperatively [28]. The evaluation included interviews, perceptual judgements of pre- versus postoperative voice characteristics, and objective acoustic measurements. Ninety 90% of the participants reported easier communication, even though 69% would prefer more volume. Unqualified recommendations for this form of treatment came from over 80% of those surveyed.

e) Nerve-Muscle Transplant

The nerve-muscle transplant is a relative newcomer on the surgical scene. Until recently, patients with bilateral vocal cord paralysis have been faced with the choice of a fairly good voice and a permanent tracheotomy, or a breathy, weak voice and adequate airway clearance. An alternative solution was proposed by Miehlke [29]. His reinnervation technique called for anastomosis of the recurrent nerve stump with the vagus. Objection to the dyssynergy which so often follows this procedure has been voiced chiefly by H. Tucker [30] whose own protocol for a nerve-muscle pedicle is described elsewhere.

·

External Laryngeal Surgery Requiring Entry Into the Vocal Tract 6

A. Thyrotomy

This chapter concerns those procedures which do require entry into the vocal tract, and one major procedure in this group is that of *thyrotomy*. Exposure of the interior of the larynx through a vertical section of the thyroid cartilage and its underlying perichondrial mucosa along the midline is the goal of a thyrotomy. It may be performed to remove benign or malignant tumors on the vocal folds or in the subglottic area. A thyrotomy can also be useful when an arytenoidectomy is performed to correct vocal fold paralysis, as well as in association with vocal fold lateralization in bilateral paralysis. Glottic stenosis may also be corrected through a thyrotomy approach and the technique finds additional application in conjunction with various functional corrections as in the plastic surgical formation of a tissue band to function as a vocal fold for a patient whose glottis has required removal.

Technique

General anesthesia is preferable, but a local agent may be utilized – and prior to the initiation of the procedure, a preliminary tracheostomy is performed. Adequate postoperative ventilation must be assured. A low, transverse collar incision is made, and the resulting skin flap is raised to the hyoid bone. The thyrohyoid membrane, thyroid cartilage, cricothyroid membrane, and cricoid cartilage all are now exposed by separating the strap muscles along the midline. Once the perichondrium overlying the thyroid cartilage is incised and reflected, the cartilage is vertically sectioned in the midline. The cricothyroid membrane is transversely incised and retracted, permitting direct visualization of the true vocal folds and of the anterior commissure. To view the interior of the larynx, one sections the laryngeal mucosa at the anterior commissure and both thyroid alae are retracted.

B. Lateral Pharyngotomy

Lateral pharyngotomy is another external laryngeal surgical approach which is often used for excision of benign tumors in the supraglottic area, malignant lesions on the lateral and posterior pharyngeal wall, and corrective procedures for subglottic stenosis.

Technique

The patient should be given general anesthesia and a tracheostomy must be performed. A transverse incision is made and the greater cornu of the hyoid bone on the side of the pharyngotomy is skeletonized, sectioned, and removed. The pharynx can be entered through the vallecula or pyriform sinus after the strap muscles at the superior border of the thyroid ala are sectioned or widely retracted. In this way, the base of the tongue, epiglottis, epiglottic fold, arytenoid, and false fold can clearly be viewed, and the lesion in question can be handled with a relatively wide surgical field, and under direct surgical vision.

C. Cricoid Split

The cricoid split is the final major procedure subserving the external laryngeal surgical approach. When subglottic stenosis is present, it may be necessary to widen the airway without immobilizing the mobile vocal folds or compromising voice production. This may be accomplished by widening the anterior portion of the cricoid using the Fearon-Cotton operation.

Techniques

A collar incision centered on the cricoid cartilage is made, exposing the laryngeal and upper tracheal cartilage. The anterior lamina of the cricoid is then split in, or near the midline and, depending on the extent of the stenosis, the split may be extended downward through the upper tracheal rings. To secure the split, a free graft of either the inferior third or the thyroid ala or a section of costal cartilage is placed between the split ends óf the cricoid lamina and tracheal rings and fixed in position with 5–0 Prolene sutures [32]. No two cases of subglottic stenosis are identical, however, and repair techniques should be adapted to each patient.

Another method utilizes the *hyoid autograft repair*. This technique calls for resecting the middle third of the hyoid bone (including periosteum) with one sternohyoid muscle attached. The cricoid cartilage overlying the stenosis is then incised, opened anteriorly, and the ends of the remaining cricoid cartilage dissected free of scar tissue. An autograft, composed of the hyoid bone and its attached muscle pedicle, is interposed between the cricoid ring edges, and sutured into place with two 28 gauge stainless steel wires. Closure is effected in layers and includes a tracheosteomy.

Hyoid arch transposition is another procedure which uses hyoid autografts [33]. Here, the stenosis is exposed by means of a median thyrotomy or a midline incision through the cricoid and anterior trachea. After scar tissue is excised, the endolarynx or endotrachea is resurfaced with a tissue graft which is sewn over a stent. Preparation for this hyoid graft consists of dissecting the suprahyoid musculature off the hyoid bone and releasing the infrahyoid membrane and musculature. The bone is then divided lateral to each lesser cornu and the hyoid segment is repositioned, and secured in place with interrupted, braided 5–0 wire sutures tied extraluminally. Whenever possible, the cricothyroid membrane and pretracheal fascia should be used to cover the graft.

D. Special Surgical Procedures

1. Lateral Arytenoid Displacement

Special procedures to be considered as component parts of the external laryngeal surgical maneuvers include four items. The first of these four is *surgery for lateral displacement of the vocal fold.* In bilateral paralysis of the vocal folds and when both folds are in the median position, an external surgical displacement of one fold, preserving its arytenoid is indicated, if the arytenoid cartilages both are mobile. Formerly these cases were treated by arytenoidectomy via a thyrotomy incision for exposure of the endolarynx. Subsequent developments, such as the King and Kelly operations and more recently, the Woodman, preserve the arytenoid cartilage while displacing it laterally. The Woodman approach requires a lateral skin incision and separation or section of the strap muscles. General anesthesia via a tracheostomy which has been created well in advance, is routine. The larynx is rotated to the opposite side by a hook or rake; the posterior edge of the thyroid lamina is reached; and the pharyngeal constrictor muscles are dissected away from it, without opening into the pharynx. Resection of a window in the thyroid lamina aids in exposing the arytenoid. The arytenoid area is palpated and the vocal process is identified. A non-absorbable suture is passed submucosally around it and sutured laterally to the thyroid lamina. Endoscopic observation is mandatory when the suture is tied so as to ensure that the resultant glottis is no less then 4 mm in width, posteriorly. Closure of surgical planes and skin follows with decannulation in a few days.

2. Functional Correction of Vocal Fold Paralysis

Surgery for functional correction of vocal fold paralysis is a newer development. The operations just described (both endoscopic or by the external route) seek to remove a vocal disorder or a respiratory encumberance by "static" means. They fix one cord so that the other can vibrate against it, or enlarge the glottis for freer respiration. However, they do leave the patient with residual vocal dysfunction. There are, however, newer procedures aimed at producing reinnervation of the paralyzed laryngeal muscles, relieving impaired laryngeal function, and restoring the voice to its fullest possible functional potential.

a) Nerve-Muscle Pedicle (Tucker) Procedure

Nerve anastomosis (suturing the cut ends of the inferior laryngeal nerve) has not yielded satisfactory results. The technique of revitalizing the paralyzed laryngeal muscles with portions of the vagus or phrenic nerves has resulted in disorderly contraction of the vocal folds (see earlier comment re: procedure). Loss of axons, neuroma formation, and Wallerian degeneration and improper reinnervation has resulted in dyssynergic vocal fold motion, unsatisfactory voice restoration, or inadequate glottal patency. Reinnervation of the posterior cricoarytenoid muscle, alone, has given better results, as proven by the restoration of abduction function in patients in whom both inferior laryngeal nerves had been destroyed. To circumvent these problems and for better preservation of, or restoration of the voice, H. Tucker developed the nerve-muscle pedicle procedure. His experiments were conducted in dogs, and in these experiments, the inferior laryngeal nerve, together with a small portion of muscle from the site where the nerve enters the larynx, were implanted into the denervated canine larynx. About 50% reinnervation was achieved two to six weeks after surgery. This procedure, in contradistinction to the previous vagal transplant, preserves the terminal nerve-muscle plaque and permits a faster recovery of function since Wallerian degeneration does not occur. Later Tucker experiments were performed in dogs in which a nerve-muscle pedicle was taken from a branch of the ansa hypoglossi (which innervates the strap muscles) and then transposed into the posterior cricoarytenoid muscle. Since electromyography shows activity of the strap muscles during inspiration, restoration of abduction was demonstrated within six weeks of the procedure.

The Tucker nerve-muscle pedicle operation has been performed in patients with bilateral vocal fold paralysis. The requirement for the procedure is that at least one arytenoid is passably mobile. Prolonged duration of the paralysis is not apparently a contraindication.

Technique   .

Through an oblique neck incision, the anterior belly of the omohyoid muscle and the jugular vein are exposed by retracting the sternocleidomastoid. The ansa hypoglossi is identified lying over the jugular vein. Anterior branches of the nerve are tested with a nerve stimulator to see if their action is on the omohyoid muscle. A block of muscle, 3–4 mm square is cut from the muscle carrying the terminal nerve-muscle plaque of the anterior branches of the ansa hypoglossi. The nerve-muscle pedicle thus created is inserted within the mass of the posterior cricoarytenoid muscle after appropriate dissection and exposure of the posterior aspect of the larynx, behind the thyroid lamina.

The nerve-muscle pedicle graft has a very sound physiological basis for its employment, and it does, when successful, obviate the troublesome loss of synergy which follows nerve-to-nerve anastomosis in many cases. In short, in Tucker's hands it is excellent. The authors feel, however, that their experience with the procedure has not always reproduced the results which Tucker was capable of obtaining, and they would thereby suggest some degree of caution in its espousal, at least until a more general concensus is obtained regarding its use.

3. Cricoarytenoid Arthrodesis

Cricoarytenoid arthrodesis is another special external laryngeal procedure. This operation is indicated in cases where the vocal fold is in abduction, the voice is weak and breathy, aspiration occurs while the patient is eating, and there is an inadequate cough reflex. The procedure repositions and fixes the arytenoid in a more medial position for proper laryngeal functioning. The preoperative and abducted position of the vocal fold may have been produced by trauma or by a dislocation of the arytenoid during intubation. The latter occurs infrequently; usually the left arytenoid is affected and it is dislocated posteriorly and laterally. If the condition is recognized early – dysphagia, hoarseness, and arytenoid swelling are the triad for diagnosis – repositioning by endoscopic manipulation is indicated. In long-standing dislocations, an external route is necessary, and the surgical approaches are similar to those previously described for arytenoid cartilage exposure. The injection of teflon, it should be noted, may also produce a similar functional result in the less dramatic case.

4. Special Indications for Lateral Pharyngotomy

Discussion and Techniques

We must finally consider in this chapter on external laryngeal surgery the *resection of benign intramural laryngeal tumors*. Cysts, especially those occurring at the vallecula, and small, limited, benign tumors elsewhere in the larynx, almost routinely cause vocal disorders and/or deficient glottal patency. Almost all of these can be removed by endoscopic procedures; but, when the size, location or nature of the mass precludes that approach, external excision via the lateral pharyngotomy approach is indicated. Cysts, as well as larger solid tumors, are included in this consideration. Anesthesia is administered through tracheostomy. A collar incision is made and laterally extended to the affected side. The strap muscles are then sectioned to secure wide exposure of the thyroid cartilage. The thyroid cartilage's periosteum is retracted, and the upper part of the lamina on the affected side is resected with careful preservation of the superior laryngeal nerve and vessels. Dissection excision of the intralaryngeal mass follows. In cases of laryngocele, the dissection should extend to the laryngeal ventricle, where the abnormality originates. Meticulous hemostasis with cautery and subsequent ligature is essential. Closure is in planes with a Penrose drain for security; decannulation is in a few days.

7*

5. Thyroid Surgery

a) Thyroid Surgery *per se*

Thyroid surgery must be considered in this chapter on external laryngeal surgery for benign conditions, since vocal deformities can and do follow thyroid abnormalities. Anatomically, the thyroid gland lies behind the infrahyoid muscles in the lower third of the neck and partially encircles the upper trachea. It consists of two ellipsoidal masses – the lateral lobes – connected anteriorly to the trachea and below the cricoid cartilage by an isthmus, the thyroid isthmus. A third pyramidal lobe arises from an adjacent portion of a lateral lobe or from the superior aspect of the isthmus and may ascend to the hyoid bone. The thyroid is attached to the cricoid cartilage with fascial bands which arise from the upper anteromedial edge of the gland and blend into the fascia overlying the cricothyroid muscle. Known as the suspensory ligaments, these ligaments cause the thyroid gland to move together with the larynx during swallowing or phonation. If strap muscle contraction is impeded on one side, tilting of the larynx (as seen through a flexible fiberoptic laryngoscope) may result, and, consequently, difficulties with voice. Accordingly, if a partial or total thyroidectomy is performed, every attempt should be made to preserve these muscles, thereby to minimize any vocal impairment.

b) Other Causes Relating to Thyroid Gland

Some benign lesions of the thyroid may also produce vocal fold paralysis as a result of pressure over the inferior laryngeal nerve. This is of course exclusive of that paralysis which is caused by thyroid malignancy, trauma or by surgical procedures on the thyroid gland itself. The mechanism is one of compression; the paralysis is usually reversible in a few weeks or months following correction of the compression. The condition is extremely rare and the diagnosis is difficult, requiring a thyroid scan and definitive diagnosis by surgical exploration itself.

c) Torticollis

Torticollis, commonly called "wry neck", is often associated with contraction of the large sternomastoid muscle contracting unilaterally, or asymmetrically and bilaterally. In addition to affecting head position, these muscle contractions can result in improper positioning of the larynx and, therefore, may etiologically be related to vocal disorders. When performing surgery to relieve sternomastoid contraction, the laryngologist must definitely consider the final larynx position, once contraction and scar formation have terminated.

d) Branchial Cleft Cysts

Branchial cleft cysts are painless swellings which develop from embryonal remnants, and whose subsequent growth produces a globular mass in the upper triangle of the neck. They may enlarge and elongate along the anterior edge of the sternocleidomastoid muscle. Therapy consists of surgical removal of the mass through an upper horizontal cervical incision. If the cyst is unusually large, it may be necessary, however, to make the incision along the anterior edge of the sternocleidomastoid muscle. The cyst should be removed intact, if possible. Care should be taken to avoid injury to various laryngeal nerves – a subject discussed in a later section.

6. Thyroglossal Duct Cysts

Thyroglossal duct cysts develop from embryonal remnants along the thyroglossal duct, itself an epithelial vestige, sometimes persisting after descent of the primordial thyroid structures. These structures originate embryologically together with the tongue base. Indeed, the normal tongue shows on the upper surface of its posterior third, a "V" shaped row of circumvallate papillae, concerned with taste. This row terminates at a point, the foramen caecum. The same indentation, the foramen caecum, marks the site at which the primordial thyroid elements began their inferior descent into the neck. Normally, the duct loses its lumen and develops into a solid epithelial cord lying either in front of, behind, or through the hyoid bone and terminating in the pyramidal lobe of the thyroid gland. Should the epithelial lining of the cord fail to degenerate, cysts and fistulas can occur, sometimes causing sensations of tension or choking in the tongue or neck.

Surgical Technique

Due to their high probability of infection, thyroglossal cysts should surgically be removed through a horizontal incision along a natural skin crease. The cyst is freed from the larynx and/or the thyrohyoid membrane and retracted upward after lateral retraction of the strap muscles has been accomplished. Because the central section of the hyoid bone is removed along with the cyst, and because of the strap muscle involvement, the surgeon must take care to secure correct laryngeal positioning during surgery.

7. Laryngocele

Laryngocele, an airfilled dilation of the appendix of the ventricle, can be classified according to the extent of dilation present. An internal laryngocele is characterized by dilation, which, remaining within the bounds of the thyroid cartilage, causes hoarseness and occasional dyspnea. An external laryngocele, however, protrudes above the thyroid cartilage and through the thyrohyoid membrane, manifesting itself as a mass in the neck. The patient presents with a full-sounding voice, again as if there were a potato in the throat.

Surgical Technique

While small internal laryngoceles may be decompressed endoscopically with a forcep, surgical resection is necessary for the large internal, and all external laryngoceles. The procedure begins with the performance of a tracheostomy. A transverse skin incision is made and the skin flap is raised to the hyoid cartilage. The strap muscles are retracted and the external laryngocele is located, mobilized and followed to the superior border of the thyroid cartilage. Subperichondrial removal of the superior third of the thyroid ala facilitates tracing the neck of the external laryngocele to its ventricular origin and permits identification and isolation of an internal laryngocele. The laryngocele is then ligated and severed. At no time is the pharynx entered and no damage is done to the superior laryngeal nerve or vessels.

Vocal Tract Surgery for Resonance Change (Excluding Hypopharynx and Larynx) 7

A. Anatomy and Discussion of Parts

It is a very well known fact that the fundamental sounds created by the vocal folds are modified in a positive or negative way by those anatomical structures which are adjacent to or distant from the larynx. In this respect, one may list virtually every structure in the upper respiratory and upper digestive systems from the hypopharynx to the nasal fossae as demonstrating an influence upon voice.

What is remarkable of this area besides its respiratory and digestive functions, is its anatomical constituent acoustical system which can be described in terms of known acoustical and physical laws. As a musical instrument, it is unique.

The fundamental vibrations created at the level of the glottis are amplified and endowed with characteristic voice qualities acoustically specific to each person by means of a series of connecting cavities which act as resonating chambers. These resonating cavities are the supraglottic inlet, the hypopharynx, oropharynx and nasopharynx, the oral cavity, the nasal fossae, and debatably, the paranasal sinuses. The size and shape of the different anatomic structures involved in this mechanism vary with the exception of the nasopharynx and paranasal sinuses. None excepting the latter two structures is a rigid structure, but a functional one which can be changed in size and tension according to the demands of sound production made by the individual concerned.

The supraglottic space produces resonance changes by approximating the two sides of the larynx and by changing the position of the epiglottis. The pharynx as a whole acts by tensing its walls, with contraction of the constrictor and accessory muscles. It also raises the larynx, thus narrowing and shortening the pharynx in its transverse and vertical diameters. The oral cavity alters resonance by motions of the tongue, lips, cheeks, and soft palate. The nasal cavity, despite rigid walls, participates in these mechanisms to some extent by widening of the nasal valvular area and the nostrils and by slow changes in the bulk of the nasal mucosa. Whether or not the paranasal sinuses contribute to resonating capacity is highly controversial and not particularly appropriate to this discussion.

Of fundamental importance in the resonating system are the actions of the soft palate and the tongue. The velum, or soft palate, functions by changing the sizes of the pharyngeal and oral cavities. Also, by contracting, it can completely exclude the nasopharynx, nasal cavities, and paranasal sinuses from the expiratory main-stream of sound flow. The tongue acts by virtue of its totally versatile mobile capacity to change in shape, volume, and position, thereby influencing the resonating qualities of both the oral cavity and the pharynx, all in addition to its fundamental role in the modulation and articulation of speech. The velum and the tongue are located precisely at the intersection of the upper respiratory and upper digestive systems, giving both those structures an important role in all the functions pertaining to voice and breathing. In professional speakers or singers, there must be changes and accomodations of the tension in the walls of these chambers to the size of the resonating cavities, all in a coordinated, balanced motion. There must be "tuning in" to the glottal vibrations. By precise modulation and articulation, there must be given to the entire system a well-accomplished integration, to result in the excellent qualities one regards as the "trained" voice.

If there is a lack of adequate coupling of these elements to each other as a result of congenital, pathologic, or postsurgical changes in their functioning or architecture, the voice quality suffers a diversion from its natural or trained characteristics. It manifests a pathologic acoustic character, dysphonia, as a consequence.

This chapter reviews some of the structures and some of their problems as they participate in comprising the vocal tract and which can produce voice disorders, and suggests surgical techniques for their correction.

B. Tonsil

1. Discussion

The tonsil is probably one of the most conspicuous of the pharyngeal contents and probably has caused the most aggregate grief of all of the pharyngeal structures. Tonsillectomy, once highly feared in the vocal professional is no longer productive of such anxiety, for if the preoperative requirements for tonsillectomy have been met (they do not differ between the professional and non-professional voice user), the surgeon's primary concern here is that of preservation of anterior and posterior tonsillar pillars. A properly executed tonsillectomy probably will not significantly alter voice, but it may enlarge the pharyngeal resonating space and thereby produce a subtle alteration in vocal resonance. There must be proper postoperative motion of the soft palate, and there must be prevention of dense, adhesive scarring. There must be preservation of the uvula as well to ensure proper mobility of the soft palate. It should be noted that when the surgeon is considering the voice of the professional, particularly that of a singer of quality, mobility of the soft palate is extremely important.

2. Voice Change After Surgery

Consideration for tonsillectomy has to be very carefully made. One cannot and must not undertake this procedure without warning the singer that there is the possibility of major vocal change and the likelihood of minor vocal change. Vocal change, if it does occur, will relate to the size of the tissue mass removed which has interfered with resonance and function, but which is nevertheless a part of the vocal tract that the individual has been trained to use and now must re-study and re-train to use comfortably and predictably. Vocal tract change after tonsillectomy may also occur from the traction of scar tissue formation. Such scarring may then produce a degree of palatal immobility. Tonsillectomy in the patient with a "valuable voice", particularly a valuable singing voice, should still be recommended with caution, but not necessarily with fear on the parts either of singer or surgeon.

C. Soft Palate

Discussion and Surgical Techniques

In the soft palate, a velopalatal insufficiency produced by a short palate, by a submucous, or by a manifest cleft palate, the voice has a characteristic hypernasality. In hypertrophy of the adenoid mass, or nasopharyngeal benign or malignant tumor, there is more or less a lack of upper resonance and the voice has a characteristic flat quality which reflects a lack in nasality. The velopalatal insufficiency created by a soft, or by a combined palatal cleft is corrected by palato-staphylorraphy, with or without associated push-back technique. Younger patients operated at two or two and one-half years of age have a better quality of voice result, to the point that the voice will often be normal or almost normal and without manifest hypernasality. Older children and adults may require, in addition, a pharyngeal flap from the posterior pharyngeal wall with its pedicle based superiorly, to improve velopharyngeal closure and speech results. The pharyngeal flap is used also when the palatal insufficiency is caused by those submucosal palatal clefts or short palates producing hypernasality. Radiological and vocal dynamic laboratory tests should be performed preoperatively to establish the nature of the vocal disorder. The surgical techniques are very specialized and will not be discussed here. Some cases, though may be improved by teflon paste injections, or by cartilage implants in the posterior pharyngeal wall, either as the sole procedure, or to complement the surgical intervention; or, as a later procedure, to further improve the results obtained by the original operation. Uncontrolled surgical excisions during tonsillectomy and contracted scars of diverse origins can produce voice disorders from their resultant cicatrization at the velopharyngeal port.

D. Nasopharynx

In a consideration of the nasopharynx, enlarged adenoids, cysts, chordomas, meningiomas, juvenile angiofibromas, or malignant tumors in the nasopharnyx all will change the quality of the voice, as their bulk impinges on the space of the cavity. Nasal respiratory insufficiency, epistaxis, etc. are usually accompanying symptoms. Surgical excision or now more rarely, X-ray therapy are the main therapeutic modalities for the management of these conditions. It is important to note that in cases of submucous palatal clefts, the adenoid mass probably should not be removed because its excision may increase hypernasality of speech. The ear surgeon may encounter the exception to this, where middle ear problems may possibly require lateral adenoidectomy with preservation of the central mass, as well as the upper pharyngeal constructor muscle mass sometimes referred to as the Ridge of Passavant.

E. Tongue

Second to the tonsil masses, probably the most conspicuously evaluated pharyngeal space occupant is the tongue. Any pathologic condition in this versatile organ will create voice disturbances. Infections and abscesses, vallecular cysts, benign tumors, such as fibromas and granular cell myoblastomas, and, finally, malignant tumors, obviously are serious considerations, and will require medical and/or surgical intervention.

1. Lingual Tonsil

Hypertrophy of the lingual tonsil may respond to medical treatment along the lines of allergic control, dietary regulation, or autogenous vaccines. If these measures fail, partial excision of the hypertrophic lingual tonsil may be considered. When this procedure is undertaken, bleeding from the tongue base can be a major consideration. Local infiltration of a dilute epinephrine and lidocaine can do much to help in this area. Recently, work with the CO_2 laser has indicated that it may also prove to be of great help here.

2. Lingual Frenulum

There are also congenital pathologic entities that will create vocal disorders, especially in modulation and articulation. Most common is the short lingual frenulum, which can be simply incised or repaired by a Z-plasty, depending on the degree of impairment and related speech disorder. "Tongue-tie" of a degree sufficient to require surgery rarely exists in infants who have enough tongue mobility to permit unimpaired nursing or sucking. The production of speech requires relatively little anterior tongue mobility, certainly not past the edge of the upper and lower teeth.

3. Macroglossia

Excessive size of the tongue – macroglossia – may impede the motions which are necessary for proper articulation. Partial resection of an excessively large tongue, following very careful studies of its articulatory effects, may improve speech as well as disorders such as tongue biting, eating problems, etc., all created by this malformation.

4. Lingual Thyroid

Some patients may have a mass at the foramen caecum of the tongue, and this mass may give rise to vocal and other disorders. The mass in question may prove, by biopsy, to be lingual thyroid gland. It is of the utmost importance that thyroid uptake and scanning studies be performed, not only to delineate the mass but also to establish that a normal thyroid gland is present in the neck. The correction of this situation – when it is confirmed that the lingual thyroid mass is the only functioning thyroid tissue in the body – consists in creating an island flap: dissecting the lingual thyroid free, in continuity with a muscular-vascular pedicle. This vascularized island flap is then transferred down into the neck through a surgically created tunnel and sutured in the desired position. In this way the patient will not be hypothyroid for life, as would be the case if the lingual thyroid were removed and no thyroid tissue existed in the neck. Where the thyroid in the neck is of sufficient size to ensure adequate functional activity, the lingual thyroid may be excised if its removal is necessary.

F. Mandible

Since the tongue is closely related to the lower jaw developmentally, congenital, developmental or traumatic disturbances of the mandible – excessive length, or its underdevelopment as in micrognathia – can produce vocal disorders. Disturbances in mandibular growth may also produce disturbances in the dental arches with faulty bite relationships. These mandibular disorders are surgically corrected by specialized procedures, which in turn are frequently combined with orthodontia further to improve the functional results.

G. Nose

1. Nasal Fossae: General Discussion of Role

The nasal fossae are also structures which influence the quality of the voice. A common observation is the hypernasality of speech which one hears at the start of a cold, followed then by denasality when the inflammatory congestion and infiltration of the mucous membrane, especially that of the turbinates with their venous lacunae, is relieved. The nasal fossa as an airway should permit an adequate intake of air, especially for the professional who must deliver a speech or sing in concert or operatic performance. It is of interest to note that nasal airway obstruction is more of a problem to the professional speaker than it is to the singer; the singer very frequently does not object to nasal obstruction except as this may produce dryness from the then-necessary mouth breathing.

However, it would be very advisable that there be nasal airway assessment prior to nasal surgery. An instrumental evaluation of airflow through the nasal airway studied both before and after mucosal shrinkage is helpful to determine the obstructive breathing component which is dependent upon organic, irreversible architectural disorder within the nose. This obstruction is in contrast to congestive, reversible disorders.

Partial nasal insufficiency requires that there be supplementary air intake through the mouth. It also implies all the adverse consequences of mouth breathing upon the throat and larynx (dryness, cold air impact, etc.) and upon the chest (bronchial irritation, lack of stimulation for deep breathing, etc.) and may take its toll in the long range, both on the individual and on his voice. Excessive airway space may also be detrimental and can be due, in some instances, to excessive surgery. An equilibrium should exist in the nasal airway between constriction and freedom to produce the optimal nasal patency. Adequate resistance to the inspiratory air flow is physiologically necessary.

2. Architectural Blockage of Airway

The pathologic conditions responsible for nasal airway obstruction and subsequent voice disorders are well known by otorhinolaryngologists and principles and procedures have long been established to correct them. The most common entities producing nasal blockage and changes in the voice are the deviated septum, hypertrophic turbinates, enlarged tails of turbinates, nasal polyps, allergy, and concha bullosa (ballooning of the bone of the middle turbinate, etc.). Relatively recently in the history of rhinology, congenital, developmental, and traumatic deformities of the nasal pyramid have been identified as producing these disturbances as well. Some of them are structural; others are disorders of function. The correction of nasal respiratory insufficiency in a professional user of the voice requires a very careful diagnostic evaluation and projection of the desired results before the surgeon should enter on a surgical procedure which might otherwise disrupt the delicate relationships already physiologically existing in the upper airway passages.

We need not describe here operations which are well detailed in current papers and treatises. We will point out only some specific elements of technique in submucous resection and rhinoplasty.

Air flow in the nasal cavity follows an arc, with its convexity rising to the upper part of the nasal cavity. One may have adequate patency in the lower part of the nose and, yet, sense nasal obstruction and lack of speaking voice resonance since the air flow does not reach the upper part of the nasal cavity in adequate amounts. The lateral alar wall may valve shut against the middle wall and produce an inspiratory obstruction.

3. Nasal Septum: Surgical Technique Considerations

The surgical correction of a septum which is deviated high in the nasal fossa, or which is too thick at the site of the septal tubercle requires special precautions. It is well known that a certain amount of cartilaginous septal strip should be left along the dorsal aspect of the septum to prevent the development of a "saddle nose." However, it must be recognized that, although the cartilaginous septum is subcutaneous caudally, when it rises superiorly and approaches the glabella, it articulates with the undersurface of the nasal bones. More posteriorly, the perpendicular plate of the ethmoid continues with the quadrilateral cartilage to the roof of the nasal cavity. Consequently, corrective resection of the septum can be carried out more superiorly in the area underneath the nasal bones, the level at which the convexity of the air flow curve becomes more marked, with a good margin of safety. Opening this area without creating the hazard of a saddle nose – since the nasal bones form a non-depressible roof to the nasal cavity – can become very important in restoring the physiology of the cavity. It should be noted that in certain cases the nasal bones may be relatively small or indented in the midline, indicating that the septal cartilage is subcutaneous in a more superior direction. Establishing this relationship will permit more precise regulation of the extent of the superior septal correction.

In those instances where the septal tubercle or the subcutaneous part of the septum is too thick, creating respiratory insufficiency in the upper nasal fossa, the mucoperichondrial linings of both sides are elevated, in septal surgery, to the place where the cartilaginous thickening is present. Since this area, in contradistinction to the situation described above, is not protected by the nasal bones, the danger of a secondary saddle nose exists. In septal resection, a dorsal aspect of the septum is thus left to support the nasal dorsum. It will be of the same size as is usually left in a standard resection; but, instead of being thick, it will be made to become thin. The upper nasal fossa by means of these maneuvers, can be opened superiorly in a more extensive fashion.

In every submucous resection, especially those which are very extensive, straight pieces of cartilage, or portions of the perpendicular plate of the ethmoid removed, are then reimplanted. If the excised fragment is thick, it is thinned, working it on a silicone cutting block with a scalpel blade. If it is deflected, it is criss-crossed until the spring of the cartilage is lessened sufficiently. If the perpendicular bony plate is deflected, it is trimmed with a small rongeur, discarding the portions which are not in a straight line, and the thin, flat, straight bone fragments are reinserted between the two fibromucous membranes. Care should be exercised to see that these pieces are not permitted to override each other, since this would create again the thickening of the septum,

Postoperatively, the final packing should be snug, although some surgeons use no packing at all, or use intranasal splints. The reimplantation of cartilage and bone has the advantage of creating a new, rigid septum which will not be moved sidewards with the changes in direction of the air flow. Such motions could occur in an extensive septal resection when only both fibromucous membranes remain, rather than in simply a septal resection alone.

4. Architecture of External Nose

We have described some elements in the correction of nasal respiratory disturbances produced by intranasal structures and, particularly, by the septum. In many instances, as mentioned before, the nasal pyramid is responsible for defective nasal physiology. Among other factors, drooping of the nasal tip, which becomes increased with age, frequently does not permit a good flow of air. In other instances, the deficiency may reside at the level of the nasal valve, a projection of the caudal portion of the upper lateral cartilage into the nasal vestibule. In this case, the deficiency is produced either by a permanent narrowing due to the thickness of the upper lateral cartilages or it may occur only during inspiration, and represents a variation of the so-called "aspiration" of the alae. The caudal ends of the upper lateral cartilages function as a check valve preventing the free inflow of air.

5. Rhinoplasty

A rhinoplasty can correct these deficiencies. Not only will it modify the esthetic appearance, but, by lifting the tip of the nose and shortening it, successful and esthetically pleasing rhinoplastic surgery will permit the air flow to follow the physiologic curve. Also, it may change the position of the upper lateral cartilages and widen the valve area. If necessary, implants of autogenous or bank cartilage or bank scleral grafts from the eye in this area may be used to help correct an excessively narrow nasal valve. The amount of dorsal excision should be carefully calculated, especially in the professional, since an incorrect – though supposedly corrective – rhinoplasty may result in further airway obstruction. Septoplasty and rhinoplasty may be performed as separate procedures or, as we prefer, as a single operation.

H. The Paranasal Sinuses

Although participation of the paranasal sinuses in vocal resonance is highly debatable, there are those who believe that these air containing cavities offer the hollow requirements for resonance. It is well known that the patient with fluid in the antrum shows a characteristic disturbance in the speaking voice which is relieved when the antral cavity is emptied. Large polyps or tumors within the sinus are sometimes considered to produce the same effect, as may pathology in the sphenoid sinus and the large posterior ethmoidal cells. It should also be noted, however, that classical singers are quite able to perform easily with fluid-filled antra, even though their sense of well-being is far short of their acoustic and resonance adequacy. Here, as noted earlier, the primary responses appear to be in speech, and not in the singing voice.

Conclusions 8

In conclusion, it is the author's hope that an overview of some of those procedures which are included in the surgical care of vocal disorders will have been furnished to an audience which would be composed of voice practitioners, therapists, teachers, speech diagnosticians, possibly the neophyte otolaryngology resident, and perhaps, and with the help of his speech therapist as guide and mentor, the interested patient himself. The effort has not been intended as a handbook to guide the operating laryngologist, nor as a surgical atlas. Rather, it has been our intention to discuss those procedures which we have now enumerated and to interpolate where we felt it appropriate, judgmental comments upon them. We have also taken this forum in which to express our views and our philosophies regarding many of the fundamental surgical exercises in the otolaryngic armentarium which is ours, both here in the United States, and in Japan as well.

But where, finally, does this leave us? If one starts again at the beginning, for example, with the Index and with the Table of Contents and considers the chapters and their subheadings specifically again and in detail, what do they tell us?

First of all, consider diagnosis, and the medical history: In all probability this single item remains as it has always been, the most illustrative, the most helpful, and the most basic of tools which is at the practitioner's disposal. Once a complete, thorough and adequate (and frequently soul-searching) history has been taken, the practitioner should have a fairly clear idea as to what the vocal problem is, as to what its genesis is, and in all likelihood, a fairly decent idea as to how it should be managed. There are, of course, specific subqualifications which do relate to occupation and environment; an endocrine history and pa-tient-habit patterns are of importance. Again, the widespread use of the anovulatory pill as a method of birth control has totally altered many parts of the laryngologist's conception of the female voice: it has been of interest to all of us to observe some of the changes in attitude, and in the practice of otolaryngology which relate specifically to this issue; many long-held concepts with respect to the effects of pre-menstrual fluid retention and edema seem now not to be quite as valid as they were a decade or so ago. The "courtesy days" which apparently were a standard inclusion in continental operatic contracts, do not appear to be as valid here when they are considered coldly and in an analytic manner.

With respect to the specific diagnostic examination procedures, there has been an amazing increase in the accuracy and in the specificity of vocal dynamics testing procedures and a corresponding increase both in the amount and in the quality of information which these procedures can yield. There has also been an increase in the amount of information available and which has become accessible to all of us through radiologic procedures, even when one considers the concept of total irradiation time and the potential for deleterious effects which are there for a subject who exceeds that irradiation exposure time: it answers increasingly more questions.

The importance of adequate medical records and specific patient records cannot too emphatically be restated, particularly in this litiginous age in which we live. No laryngologist should now propose and undertake corrective surgery upon the larynx of an individual who presents to him with a complaint referrable to voice quality or voice function, without obtaining preoperative recordings of the voice of that patient, both for his own education and for that of the patient.

There should be noted the ever-increasing role of naso-laryngoscopy with a flexible fiberoptic laryngoscope, particularly when this instrumentation is combined with the television camera and permanent recording on television cassette tape. With this instrumentation, remarkable things occur and appear. It is impossible for the viewer to encompass all of the specific movements of the aggregate components of laryngeal anatomy at one viewing of the image. Those of us who have been privileged to work with a television camera attached to the naso-laryngoscope are unanimous in our enthusiasm for the assistance it provides in diagnosis and in documentation: as a means for recording the preoperative status of a presurgical patient, it is unparallelled. As a teaching instrument for the laryngologic surgeon, for the speech and/or voice therapist and for the patient, it is of inestimable value.

Mirror laryngoscopy still retains its position as the basic tool used in office laryngology, and its position as the basis from which virtually all laryngeal diagnoses proceed. In this same context, use of the angulated fixed fiberoptic laryngoscope will probably increase and be of widening value to the speech therapist, requiring as it does nothing, or at best little in the way of topical anesthesia.

Apropos indirect laryngoscopy: Almost the only surgical technique which now would be permissible in the average medical center if the surgeon were to use only mirror laryngoscopy for his view of the larynx, would be the technique of teflon injection for the repositioning of a paralyzed vocal fold. There have been, and will always be certain individuals who are highly skilled in the use of mirror laryngoscopy as a primary means of visualizing the larynx for specific surgical procedures. This is not, however, the usual case, and one suspects that these individual circumstances will lessen even more as time passes.

More and more procedures will be done under general anesthesia for direct laryngoscopy, providing as it does, the immobile operating field which is necessary for the performance of adequate microlaryngeal surgical procedures. Any time that it is possible to undertake a surgical procedure adequately and successfully via the endolaryngeal route one should certainly do so. This is helpful with respect to cost, with respect to morbidity and with respect to disturbance of overall physiology. There is little argument that the endolaryngeal management of the commoner lesions, nodes and polyps and papillomata, for example, is to be preferred. There has also been an explosive growth in the indications for use of laser surgery via the endolaryngeal route and it is strongly to be anticipated that a similar trend will continue.

With respect to external laryngeal surgery for benign *vocal* conditions, this is a relatively new idea; at least at this particular moment, it is not one which commands universal acceptance in the English-speaking community. There are unarguable advantages to surgical approaches via this route and the potential for minimizing mucosal disruption and subsequent scarring of the vocal folds is undeniable. These procedures are not universally accepted, nor applied, nor are they universally employed. While one admits readily of their theoretical advantages, one is equally aware that there is not a large number of surgeons correctly and appropriately trained to undertake them now current. Training for this sort of surgery is not now generally widely available to many laryngology residents.

Surgical procedures for branchial cleft cysts, thyroglossal duct cysts and their like have been fairly constant for some years and it is anticipated that this will remain the case. It will be, however, interesting to see what does occur during the 1980's with respect to another external laryngeal surgical procedure: specifically that of Dr. H. Tucker with respect to nerve-muscle pedicle grafting for the reinnervation of a paralyzed vocal fold. This procedure does have an adequate, accurate and sound physiologic basis. As of the early 1980's, it does not appear to be generally accepted in many of the teaching centers.

If one excludes surgical procedures on the hypopharynx and larynx and considers only surgical procedures on pharyngeal structures, there has been relatively little change in the preceding years. The entire subject would appear to be likely to remain a static one.

With respect to the entire subject of vocal tract surgery for benign conditions, one could do worse than to consider again a statement made in the opening passages of this work. Considering the management of a patient with a specific vocal tract problem "in short, there should ideally be a team; a team consisting of a good speech therapist–diagnostician who maintains close rapport with the patient, an involved laryngologist who has his wits about him and his diagnostic acumen sharpened, plus a strongly motivated patient who comprehends his participation in the overall scheme of things as well as his diagnosis and prognosis. This team then ought to do fairly well with the satisfactory management, with the satisfactory solution of problems besetting the subject with most of more common voice disorders. A requirement of surgery often means that somewhere along the line one of the team members has faltered, has misdiagnosed, has lost enthusiasm or momentum." One could finally, but profitably reconsider again an aphorism of one of our giants in contemporary architecture, Mies van der Rohe, for it says also a great deal about what we consider to be a basic truth applicable to vocal tract surgery for benign lesions as well: "Less is more."

References

1. Gould, W. J.: The Gould laryngoscope. Trans. Am. Acad. Ophthalmol. Otol. 77, 139–141 (1973).
2. Dedo, H. H., Urrea, R. O., Lawson, L.: Intracordal injection of teflon in treatment of 135 patients with dysphonia. Ann. Otol. Rhinol. Laryngol. 82, 661–667 (1973).
3. Rubin, H. J.: Misadventures with injectable polytef (teflon). Arch. Otolaryngol. 101, 114–116 (1975).
4. Lewy, R. B.: Experience with vocal cord injection. Ann. Otol. Rhinol. Laryngol. 85, 440–450 (1976).
5. Brunings, W.: Die Defekte. In: Laryngoskopie, Bronchoskopie und Ösophagoskopie: Ein Handbuch für die Technik der direkten okularen Methoden. Wiesbaden: Bergmann. 1970.
6. Kleinsasser, O., et al.: Microlaryngoscopy and endolaryngeal microsurgery. London: W. B. Saunders. 1969.
7. Killian, G.: Suspension laryngoscopy – a modification of the direct method. Trans. 3rd Internat. Laryngolog. Congr., Berlin, Germany, (Part II) Transactions P. 12, 1911.
8. Jackson, C.: Peroral endoscopy and laryngeal surgery. St. Louis, Mo.: Laryngoscope Co. 1915.
9. Holinger, P.: An hour-glass anterior commissure laryngoscope. Laryngoscope 70, 1570–1571 (1960).
10. Jako, G.: Laryngoscope for microscopic observation, surgery, and photography. Arch. Otolaryngol. 91, 196–199 (1970).
11. Dedo, H. H.: A fiberoptic anterior commissure laryngoscope for use with the operating microscope. Trans. Am. Acad. Ophthalmol. Otol. 82, 91–92 (1976).
12. Demeester, T. R., Skinner, D. B., Evans, R. H., Benson, D. W.: Local nerve block anesthesia for peroral endoscopy. Ann. Thoracic Surg. 24, 278–283 (1977).
13. Calcaterra, T. C., House, J.: Local anesthesia for suspension microlaryngoscopy. Ann. Otol. Rhinol. Laryngol. 85, 71–73 (1976).
14. Carden, E., Becker, G., Hamood, H.: Percutaneous jet ventilation. Ann. Otol. Rhinol. Laryngol. 85, 652–655 (1976).
15. Carden, E., Ferguson, G. B., Crutchfield, W.: A new silicone elastomer tube for use during microsurgery on the larynx. Ann. Otol. Rhinol. Laryngol. 83, 360–364 (1974).
16. Urban, G. D., jr.: Laryngeal microsurgery without intubation. South Med. T. 69, 828–830 (1976).
17. Norton, M. D., Strong, M. S., Snow, J. C., Vaughan, C. W., Kripke, B. J.: Endotracheal intubation and Venturi (jet) ventilation for laser microsurgery of the larynx. Ann. Otol. Rhinol. Laryngol. 85, 656–663 (1976).

18. Gould, W. J.: A new reversible action laryngeal forceps. Trans. Am. Acad. Ophthalmol. Otol. 77, 1137–1138 (1973).
19. Miller, D.: Cryosurgery as a modality in treatment of carcinoma of the larynx. Laryngoscope 85, 1281–1285 (1975).
20. Hong, S. W., Silverskin, H., Sadeghee, S.: The effect of cryosurgery on the canine and human larynx. Laryngoscope 87, 1079–1085 (1977).
21. Vaughn, C. W., Strong, M. S., Jako, G. T.: Laryngeal carcinoma: Transoral treatment utilizing the CO_2 laser. Am. J. Surg. 136, 490–493 (1978).
22. Kirchner, F. A.: Laryngeal structure following microcauterization. Laryngoscope 85, 797–805 (1975).
23. Strong, M. S., Vaughn, C. W., Copperband, S. R., Healy, G. B., Clemente, M. A. C. P.: Recurrent respiratory papillomatoses: management with CO_2 laser. Ann. Otol. Rhinol. Laryngol. 85, 508–516 (1976).
24. Andrews, A.: Verbal communication.
25. Bloch, C. S., Gould, W. J.: Vocal therapy in lieu of surgery for contact granuloma: A case report. J. Speech Hear Disord. 39, 478–485 (1974).
26. Dedo, H. H.: Recurrent laryngeal nerve section for spastic dysphonia. Ann. Otol. Rhinol. Laryngol. 85, 451–459 (1976).
27. Brodnitz, F. S.: Spastic dysphonia. Ann. Otol. Rhinol. Laryngol. 85, 210–214 (1976).
28. Izdebski, K.: Personal communication.
29. Miehlke, A.: Rehabilitation of vocal cord paralysis. Arch. Otolaryngol. 100, 431–441 (1974).
30. Tucker, H. M.: Human laryngeal reinnervation. Laryngoscope 86, 769–779 (1976).
31. Isshiki, N., Okamura, H., Ishikawa, T.: Thyroplasty type I. (lateral compression) for dysphonia due to vocal cord paralysis or atrophy. Acta Otolaryngol. 80, 465–473 (1975).
32. Fearon, B., Cinnamond, M.: Surgical correction of subglottic stenosis of the larynx: Clinical results of Fearon-Cotton operations. J. Otolaryngol. 5, 475–478 (1976).
33. Druck, N. S., et al.: Hyoid arch transposition. Trans Am. Acad. Ophthalmol. Otol. 82, 175–187 (1976).
34. von Leden, H.: Laryngology: from Galen to Garcia. Otolaryngology Head Neck Surg. 90, 226–232 (1982).
35. Garcia, M.: Physiological observations on the human voice. Proc. R. Soc. (Lond.) 7, 399 (1855).
36. Leonardo da Vinci: Quarderni d'Anatomia, c 1500.
37. Ferrein, A.: La formation de la voix de l'homme. Mém. de l'Acad. Roy. de Sci. 1741, 409.
38. Jako, G. J.: Laser surgery of the vocal cords. An experimental study with carbon dioxide laser on dogs. Laryngoscope 82, 2204–2216 (1972).
39. Polanyi, T. G., Bredemeier, H. C., Davis, T. W., jr.: A CO_2 laser for surgical research. Med. Biol. Eng. 8, 541 (1970).
40. Goldman, L., Rockwell, R. J.: Lasers in Medicine. New York: Gordon and Breach. 1971.
41. Mihashi, S., Jako, G. J., Incze, J., Strong, M. S., Vaughan, G. W.: Laser surgery in otolaryngology: Interaction of CO_2 laser in soft tissue. Ann. N. Y. Acad. Sci. 267, 263–294 (1976).
42. Yahr, W. Z., Strully, K. T.: Blood vessels anastomosis by laser and other biomedical applications. J. Assoc. Adv. Med. Instrum. 1, 28 (1966).
43. Fourcin, A.: Laryngographic examination of vocal fold vibration. In: Ventilatory and Phonatory Control Systems (Wyke, B., ed.). Oxford: 1974.
44. Reed, V. W.: The electroglottograph in voice teaching. In: Tenth Symposium Care of the Professional Voice, Part II (Lawrence, V., ed.). New York: The Voice Foundation. 1981.
45. Teaney, D.: The electroglottograph as a clinical tool for the observation and analysis of vocal fold vibration. In: Tenth Symposium Care of the Professional Voice, Part II (Lawrence, V., ed.). New York: The Voice Foundation. 1981.
46. Galenus, C.: De usu partium corporis humani; De dissectione nervorum; De locis affectis; De arte medica; De anatomia admin; De anatomia vivor. Second century AD.
47. Vesalius, A.: De Humani Corporis Fabrica. Basel: 1542.
48. Faaborg-Andersen, K., Yanagihara, N., von Leden, H.: Vocal pitch and intensity regulation. Arch. Otolaryngol. 85, 448–454 (1967).

49. Rubin, H. J., Hills, B., Lecover, M., Vennard, W.: Vocal intensity, subglottic pressure and air flow relationship in singers. Folia phoniat. *19*, 393–413 (1967).

50. Bunch, M.: Dynamics of the Singing Voice. (Disorders of Human Communication, Vol. 6.) Wien-New York: Springer. 1982.

51. Tucker, H. M.: Surgery for Phonatory Disorders. New York: Churchill. 1981.

52. Dickey, R. P.: ACOG Seminar in family planning. Medical Science, May 1967.

53. Sataloff, R. T.: Professional Singers: The science and art of clinical care. Amer. J. Otolaryngol. *2*, 251 (1981).

54. Brodnitz, F.: Medical care for the professional voice (panel). In: Transcripts of the Eigth Symposium, Care of the Professional Voice (Lawrence, V., ed.). New York: The Voice Foundation. 1979.

55. Proctor, D. F.: Breathing, Speech and Song. Wien-New York: Springer. 1980.

56. Kunze, L. E.: Evaluation of methods of estimating subglottal air pressure. J. Sp. Hear. Res. *7*, 151–164 (1964).

57. Hirano, M.: Clinical Examinations of Voice. (Disorders of Human Communications, Vol. 5.) Wien-New York: Springer. 1981.

58. Kakita, Y., Hirano, M., Matsushita, H., Hiki, S., Imaizumi, S.: Differentiation of laryngeal diseases using acoustical analysis. Pract. Otol. (Kyoto) *70*, 729–739 (1977b).

59. Isshiki, N., Okamura, H., Tanabe, M., Morimoto, M.: Differential diagnosis of hoarseness. Folia phoniat. *21*, 9–19 (1969).

60. Squires, L. F.: Fundamentals of Radiology. Commonwealth Fund. Cambridge: Harvard University Press. 1982.

61. Andrews, A. H., Moss, H. W.: Experiences with the carbon dioxide laser in the larynx. Ann. Otol. Rhinol. Larynx. *83*, 462–470 (1974).

62. Jako, G. J.: Laser surgery of the vocal cords. Laryngoscope (St. Louis) *82*, 2204–2216 (1972).

63. Mishashi, S., Jako, G. J., Incze, J., Strong, M. S., Vaughan, C. W.: Laser surgery in otolaryngology: interaction of CO_2 laser and soft tissue. Ann. N. Y. Acad. Sci. *267*, 263–294 (1976).

64. Strong, M. S., Jako, G. J.: Laser surgery in the larynx. Ann. Otol. Rhinol. Larynx. *81*, 791–798 (1972).

65. Isshiki, N., Morita, H., Okamura, H., Hiramoto, M.: Thyroplasty as a new phonosurgical technique. Acta Otolaryngol. *78*, 451–457 (1974).

66. Isshiki, N., Okamura, H., Ishikawa, T.: Thyroplasty type I (lateral compression for dysphonia due to vocal cord paralysis or atrophy. Acta Otolaryngol. *80*, 465–473 (1975).

67. Isshiki, N.: Recent advances in phonosurgery. Folia phoniat. *32*, 119–154 (1980).

68. Isshiki, N.: Functional surgery of the larynx (in Japanese). Special Report Jap. Soc. Otorhinolar. ENT. Dept. Kyoto Univ. Kyoto *1977*, 1–207.

69. Gurr, E.: Untersuchungen zur Feststellung der Lage des Stimmbandes am uneröffneten Kehlkopf. Z. Laryng. Rhinol. *27*, 71 (1948).

70. Snell, C.: On the function of the cricoarytenoid joints in the movements of the vocal cords. Proc. Kon. Nederl. Acad. Wet. *50*, 1370–1381 (1947).

71. Sonesson, B.: Die functionelle Anatomie des Cricoarytenoidgelenkes. Z. für Anatomie und Entwicklungsgeschichte *121*, 292–303 (1959).

72. Frable, M. A.: Computation of motion at the cricoarytenoid joint. Arch. Otolaryngol. *73*, 73–78 (1961).

73. von Leden, H., Moore, P.: The mechanics of the cricoarytenoid joint. Arch. Otolaryngol. *73*, 541–550 (1961).

74. Hurst, W. B.: Percutaneous injection of a vocal cord with Teflon. J. Laryng. Otol. *86*, 633–635 (1972).

75. Payr: Plastik am Schildknorpel zur Behebung der Folgen einseitiger Stimmbandlähmung. Dtsch. med. Wschr. *43*, 1265–1270 (1915).

76. Meurman, Y.: Operative mediofixation of the vocal cord in complete unilateral paralysis. Archs. Otolar. *55*, 544–553 (1952).

77. Opheim, O.: Unilateral paralysis of the vocal cord. Operative treatment. Acta Otolaryngol. *45*, 226–230 (1955).

78. Şawashima, M., Tolsuka, G., Kobayashi, T., Hirose, H.: Surgery for hoarseness due to unilateral vocal cord paralysis. Archs. Otolar. *87*, 289–294 (1968).
79. Kamer, F. M., Som, M. L.: Correction of the traumatically abducted vocal cord. Archs. Otolar. *95*, 6–9 (1972).
80. Isshiki, N., Tanabe, M., Sawada, M.: Arythenoid adduction for unilateral vocal cord paralysis. Archs. Otolar. *104*, 555–558 (1978).
81. Isshiki, N., Ishikawa, T.: Diagnostic value of tomography in unilateral vocal cord paralysis. Laryngoscope *86*, 1573–1578 (1976).
82. Isshiki, N.: Phonosurgery to change vocal pitch. HNO-Praxis (Leipzig) *6*, 179–180 (1981).
83. Isshiki, N., Taira, T., Tanabe, M.: Surgical alteration of the vocal pitch. J. Otolaryngol. (Toronto) *12*, 335–340 (1983).
84. Saito, S.: Phonosurgery – basic study on the mechanism of phonation and endolaryngeal microsurgery (in Japanese). Otologica (Fukuoka) *23*, suppl. , 171–384 (1977).
85. Isshiki, N., Tanabe, M., Ishizaka, K., Broad, D.: Clinical significance of asymmetrical vocal cord tension. Ann. Otol. Rhinol. Laryngol. *86*, 58–66 (1977).

Recommended Reading List for Cordal Injection

Arnold, G. E.: Vocal rehabilitation of paralytic dysphonia. Archs. Otolar. *76*, 358–368 (1962).
Arnold, G. E.: Alleviation of aphonia or dysphonia through intrachordal injection of teflon paste. Ann. Otol. Rhinol. Laryngol. *72*, 384–395 (1963).
Boedts, D., Roels, H., Klugskens, P.: Laryngeal tissue response to Teflon. Archs. Otolar. *86*, 110 (1967).
Brünings, W.: Über eine neue Behandlungsmethode der Rekurrenslähmung. Verh. Ver. dtsch. Lar. *18*, 18, 93–151 (1911).
Dedo, H. H., Urrea, R. D., Lawson, L.: Intracordal injection of Teflon in treatment of 135 patients with dysphonia. Laryngoscope (St. Louis) *83*, 1293–1299 (1973).
Fritzell, B., Hallen, O., Sundberg, J.: Evaluation of teflon injection procedures for paralytic dysphonia. Folia phoniat. *26*, 414–421 (1974).
Fukuda, H.: Vocal rehabilitation by injectable silicone. (In Japanese.) Jap. J. Otorhinolar. (Tokyo) *73*, 1506–1526 (1970).
Goff, W. F.: Teflon injection for vocal cord paralysis. Archs. Otolar. *90*, 124–128 (1969).
Harris, H. E., Hawk, W. A.: Laryngeal injection of teflon paste. Report of a case with postmortem study of the larynx. Archs. Otolar. *90*, 194–197 (1969).
Hirano, M.: Phonosurgery, basic and clinical investigations. (In Japanese.) Otologica (Fukuoka) *21*, suppl. 1, 239–442 (1975).
Hurst, W. B.: Percutaneous injection of a vocal cord with Teflon. J. Lar. Otol. *86*, 633–635 (1972).
Kirchner, F. R.: Toledo, P. S., Svoboda, D. J.: Studies of the larynx after teflon injection. Archs. Otolar. *83*, 350–354 (1966).
Kresa, Z., Rems, J., Wichterle, O.: Hydron gel implants in vocal cords. Acta Otolaryngol. *76*, 360–365 (1973).
von Leden, H., Yanagihara, N., Werner-Kukuk, E.: Teflon in unilateral vocal cord paralysis: preoperative and postoperative function studies. Archs. Otolar. *85*, 666–674 (1967).
Lewy, R. B.: Glottic reformation with voice rehabilitation in vocal cord paralysis: the injection of teflon and tantalum. Laryngoscope (St. Louis) *73*, 547–555 (1963).
Lewy, R. B.: Responses of laryngeal tissue to granular teflon in situ. Archs. Otolar. *83*, 355–359 (1966).
Lewy, R. B.: Experience with vocal cord injection. Ann. Otol. Rhinol. Laryngol. *85*, 440–450 (1976).
Riska, T. B., Lauerma, S., Siirala, U.: Vocal cord paralysis treated with teflon implantation. Acta Otolaryngol. *75*, 357–376 (1973).
Rontal, E., Rontal, M., Rolnick, M.: The use of spectrograms in the evaluation of vocal cord injection. Laryngoscope (St. Louis) *85*, 47–56 (1975).
Rubin, H. J.: Intracordal injection of silicon in selected dysphonias. Archs. Otolar. *81*, 604–607 (1965).

Rubin, H. J.: Misadventures with injectable polytef (Teflon). Archs. Otolar. *101*, 114–116 (1975).

Saito, S.: Phonosurgery – basic study on the mechanism of phonation and endolaryngeal microsurgery. (In Japanese.) Otologica (Fukuoka) *23*, suppl. 1, 171–384 (1977).

Stephens, C. B., Arnold, G. E., Stone, J. W.: Larynx injected with Polytef paste. Archs. Otolar. *102*, 432–435 (1976).

Stone, J. W., Arnold, G. E.: Human larynx injected with Teflon paste. Archs. Otolar. *86*, 98–109 (1967).

Suzuki, Y., Murakami, Y., Hayashi, Y., Utsumi, M., Saito, S., Fukuda, H., Ogino, M., Ogata, K.: Application of silastic to unilateral vocal cord paralysis and vocal cord atrophy. J. Jap. broncho-esoph. Soc. *19*, 151–158 (1968).

Westhues, M.: Die endoskopische Behandlung der Stimmlippenlähmungen. Z. Laryng. Rhinol. Otol. *50*, 558–562 (1971).

Subject Index

Disorders of Human Communication

Edited by **Godfrey E. Arnold, Fritz Winckel, Barry D. Wyke**

Executive Editor: **Barry D. Wyke**

**Springer-Verlag
Wien New York**

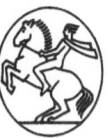